Health after Forty

Health is Wealth - Read your way to Both

DR. GEETA SUNDAR
MD

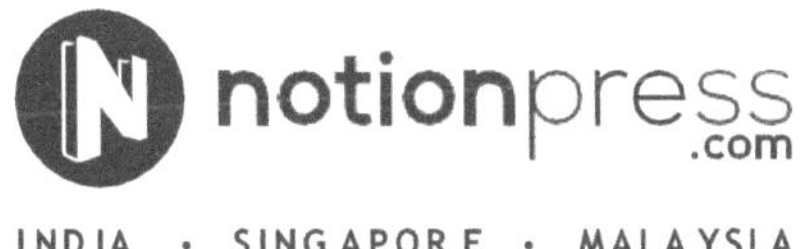

INDIA · SINGAPORE · MALAYSIA

Health after Forty

DR. GEETA SUNDAR
MD

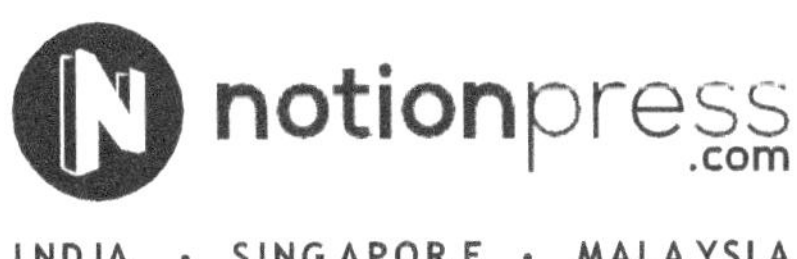

Health After Forty

Forward I

Health after Forty, by Dr. Geeta Sundar M.D., is a good guidebook for everyone who is conscious of health.

For me, health is like a river where the water flows unendingly, moment-to-moment and where one cannot dip in the same water again. It is a state where one experiences the reality beyond the elemental. Particularly after the age of forty, emotional upheavals, economic stress and environmental influences are quick to affect one's physical and mental health.

Dr. Geeta Sundar explains in her book, about the change in life, that brings physical disturbances and mental discontentment. With her knowledge of other 'pathies' she shows the way of leading a satisfactory life. She deals with exercise at the end, by introducing some simple but basic use of the structural or anatomical sheath of the body, to obtain relief.

The author has mentioned dos and don'ts in nutrition, detailing what balanced food is and how to eat with reverence. This is enough to know how much you have to value your food.

As the adage goes, "As you sow, so shall you reap" The health adage is, "As you eat, so shall you become."

The author also explains the symptoms of common

ailments that afflict a human being and shows the ways of prevention and basic movements for relief.

Health has to be earned by discipline. It cannot be purchased in a bazaar.

Dr. Geeta Sundar, with her body knowledge has shown ways of keeping the vital organs the physiological sheath healthy.

Dr. Geeta Sundar in her book has given good hints for leading a healthy life and I feel that this is a good guide for health.

YOGACHARYA B.K.S. IYENGAR

Ramamani Iyengar Memorial Yoga Institute, Pune

Forward II

I have gone through Health after Forty written by Dr Geeta Sundar, MD, Consultant Physician.

It is an excellent and succinct narration of the ailments one comes across after forty years of age and has many useful tips on how to face these problems with wisdom. The book covers almost every conceivable aspect of health. As one grows older one is bound to face one or the other of these problems and the book makes an excellent-home guide, despite its being so short, and the subject so vast.

I can commend the book to all those who are edging towards forty and hope they will benefit by following the many useful tips in the book.

TN SESHAN

IAS Former Chief Election Commissioner of India

Acknowledgments

This book is a result of the collective efforts of many hands & minds, that have helped, encouraged, inspired, & guided me from its conception to its culmination.

Dr. Geeta Sundar

✦ ✦ ✦ ✦

Introduction

"Let us endeavour so to live that when we die,
even the undertaker will be sorry"

- Mark Twain

There are two ways of aging - the wrong way, best illustrated by the old man, who was "A sitting on the gate" (by Lewis Carroll) –from "Alice in wonderland,"

"Whose look was mild, whose speech was low,

Whose hair was whiter than snow?

Whose face was very like crow,

With eyes like cinders all aglow,

Who seemed distracted by his woe,

Who racked his body to and fro,

And muttered mumblingly low,

As if his mouth were full of dough"

Here you get the typical pessimistic person who has *given in* to old age and shows it in his appearance and attitude. Contrast this with another old man as in "You are old father William" (also by Lewis Carroll, from the same book)

"You are old father William" the young man said,

"And your hair has become very white;

And yet you incessantly stand on your head –

Do you think at your age it is right?"

"In my youth", father William replied to his son

"I feared it might injure the brain;

But now that I'm perfectly sure I have none,

Why I do it again and again".

"You are old ", said the youth "as I mentioned before,

And have grown uncommonly fat;

Yet you turned a back somersault in at the door –

Pray what is the reason of that? "

"In my youth "said the sage, as he shook his grey locks,

"I kept all my limbs very supple, by the use of this
ointment – one shilling the box

Allow me to sell you a couple?"

"You are old " said the youth, and "your jaws are too weak

For anything tougher than suet;

Yet you finished the goose, with the bones and the beak –

Pray how do you manage to do it?"

"In my youth" said his father, "I took to the law

And argued each case with my wife;

And the muscular strength which it gave to my jaw,

Has lasted the rest of my life".

"You are old" said the youth, "one would hardly suppose

That your eye was as steady as ever;

Yet, you balanced an eel on the end of your nose –

What made you so awfully clever?" "I've answered three questions, and that is enough" said his father;

"Don't give yourself airs!

Do you think I can listen all day to such stuff?

Be off, or I'll kick you downstairs!"

The old man sitting on the gate was just *sitting;* and also he was *wizened, "distracted by his woe"* and *"looked like a crow".* On the other hand, the lovable old father William has found the right prescription to age correctly by *"turning somersaults, balancing eels on his nose"* and *"eating the goose with the bones and the beak".* He also knows how to *"use his ointments",* and the benefits of exercising his body, to keep *"kicking fit!"*

This is what this book is all about - the right way to age, and to equip the reader with the knowledge required to guide him through the remaining part of his life, also to have a positive outlook, and not to give in to his woes. The examples of people like "Khush"want Singh and Ashok Kumar come to mind of people who retained the twinkle in their eyes and an abundant zest for life, even into their eighties, both having wound up their innings. Victor Hugo once consoled a friend despondent at having turned fifty thus—"You should rejoice my friend that you have escaped the old age of youth and have entered the youth of old age!" Charles Colton has also very aptly remarked, "It is bad when the mind survives the body, worse when the body survives the mind, but when both survive our spirits, our hope and our health, it is worst of all!"

At forty, we are like the Greek God Janus who looks both to the past and the future, (January is therefore named after him). Behind us is the life we have lived to the full, including birth, infancy, education, career, marriage and children – each following the other almost without a pause, leaving us no time to take stock of our lives. Ahead lies the future, which could be another forty years or more, given the general increase in longevity.

There are also widespread misconceptions about health, which at times can prove outright dangerous so it is important to equip ourselves with scientific knowledge, to be able to navigate successfully, the remaining years of our lives.

Most diseases originate from the stomach, so we discuss **nutrition,** its dos and don'ts and especially when to take, and when to avoid nutritional supplements since any **tonic** taken indiscriminately and over prolonged periods, can turn into a **toxin**.

There is a lot of controversy and confusion regarding **fats** and **oils** – whether to take saturated or unsaturated, refined or unrefined, which oil to use as cooking medium etc. An attempt has been made in this book to demystify this important topic.

Bowel problems, both constipation and diarrhoea are common in a forty plus individual, and we should know how to handle them without harming ourselves, as also another burning problem called **hyperacidity**. Complaints of **eyes, teeth, nose** and **ears become** frequent as we grow older, and it is useful to know how to take care of these organs, which have served us well, and with proper care, will continue to do so for many years to come.

An aging **skin** needs extra care, and some of you may want to know about the latest advances in **cosmetic techniques,** so a few of these have been included.

We all experience **headache** and **giddiness** sometime or the other, and we should know their causes and methods of treatment.

Bones and **joints** also need special attention, as we grow older; and hence their care, as also management of **arthritis, spondylitis and osteoporosis** has been included.

With the kind of stressful life that we lead, problems of **mind** are becoming increasingly common. It cannot be emphasised enough that people with mental problems should be encouraged to come forward and get them treated, as with newer therapies, it is possible to carry on their routine activities and to be a part of the mainstream. There is also a need for changing public opinion, to prevent ostracization of these patients, who are no different from those having diseases of the body. . Since **stress** can also cause many physical problems, it is important to know how to handle it with attitudinal changes & other methods. **Diabetes, hypertension, obesity and heart disease** have reached almost epidemic proportions in urban adult population and the importance of prevention, need for proper control and management of these conditions in order to avoid complications, especially with **life style modification**, cannot be stressed enough.

Another frequently seen problem in a forty plus is that of **Thyroid**, & one must know what signs to look out for, so that this problem is detected early, since many times, weakness attributed to aging, is actually due to thyroid deficiency. **Asthma and allergy** are also very common nowadays and their proper management, especially preventive measures should be properly understood.

Some complaints like **fever pain & swelling**, are good for us, why they should not be haphazardly suppressed, has been emphasised in the chapter dealing with them, but if there is one fear that all forty plus have, it is the fear of **paralysis** and becoming dependent on others, so the knowledge of why it occurs, as also how to prevent and manage it, is very essential.

Incidence of **cancer** is also increasing with rise in stress and pollution, but with early diagnosis, it can be curable, and hence correct methods of self-examination of our bodies and importance of regular medical check-ups have been covered.

Two other common anxieties as we grow older are those of **menopause,** and fear of **sexual decline**. Both these problems need to be put in their proper perspective, including pros and cons of newer treatment modalities.

Some newer **investigative & surgical techniques** have been explained.

Exercise is of tremendous benefit in preventing disease and maintaining health and with that end, a few simple exercises have been included for most problems, which if practiced regularly, will go a long way in keeping us fit and alert in our life after forty.

Patients also need to be made aware of their **rights,** and if they exercise them judiciously, incidences of malpractice complaints against doctors will come down. Also at least one member of each family should be trained in **first aid** and some basic knowledge for everyone is useful as it can save lives in an emergency. **Medical check up** if done regularly will help in early detection and better management of disease so, to that end, a list of suggested tests in men & women has been included. What happens inside the **aging body** has been explained in the penultimate chapter. Finally all of us have to die one day, and I am sure everyone would like to understand about **death** and the current status of **Euthanasia or mercy killing** which has been dealt with in the final chapter.

A conscious attempt has been made to keep the language simple, but wherever technical terms have been included, explanations have been provided. The book covers all aspects of aging and the common ailments that are likely to occur, after forty till death. The exercise-pictures especially have been painstakingly created and a conscious attempt has been made to provide illustrations wherever needed. Having some literary pretensions, I have tried to make the book interesting with a few anecdotes, some of my amateur poetry, quotes, and case histories.

TAKE HOME MESSAGE

We have all come into this world with a certain set of handicaps & advantages. It is up to us, to downplay the former & highlight the latter, so as to achieve, what may be called a "peaceful death", or a smooth transition from one life to the other. This can be achieved by a four-pronged approach of **exercise, good nutrition, proper disease management & maintaining mental balance.** A beginning can be made at any age, so the strong take home message of this book is -

- it's never too late to change to a healthy lifestyle!

Happy Reading!

✦ ✦ ✦

Contents

PART – II

Problems which can affect Many of us

PART – III

Problems which may affect only Some of us

PART IV

Some useful Health related Knowledge

Contents

Part – I

Problems which Affect Most of us

1

Hyperacidity
a Burning Problem

A rare breed nowadays, is a forty plus individual who has never suffered from heartburn. Hyperacidity is becoming increasingly common, due to sedentary lifestyle and fast food culture.

We must understand that acid is *normally* present in our stomach and *aids* in digestion; however, when we irritate and abuse our digestive systems, we transform this useful ally into a ferocious monster, needing veterinary doses of antacids to suppress it. The answer lies in preventing such episodes from developing by trying to avoid anything or any situation, which can trigger hyperacidity.

WHAT ARE THE CAUSES OF HYPERACIDITY?

Acid secretion can increase due to some infections, mental stress, smoking, chewing tobacco, intake of alcohol, strong tea and coffee, food which is eaten too hot or too spicy, non vegetarian foods (which are all acidic) and foods which are difficult to digest - like fried foods, non-vegetarian foods, ground nuts, (pea-nuts) cashew nuts, pistachios, whole pulses and lentils, cheese, etc., and lastly sour foods being naturally acidic, also increase acid levels in stomach.

HOW CAN WE PREVENT ATTACKS?

To prevent attacks we must avoid all these triggers. Also, eat slowly, & chew food thoroughly, as it aids in digestion thus reducing the need for acid secretion. *All greens are alkaline* and neutralise acid; so obviously, green vegetables (cooked and salads) are good for acidity. Four hourly small meals (avoiding fasting and feasting) are advocated, as is sweetened, cold rose milk (not chilled) during an attack. And remember this axiom – avoid hurry, curry and worry!

There was a gentleman called Alexis St. Martin, who suffered a gunshot wound which led to a healed open passage from his skin to his stomach. Doctors could feed him all sorts of things and directly observe (by means of a pipe and torch) their effect on the stomach. Now of course, we have gastro- scopes through which all hyperacidity patients should be shown how wrong eating habits harm their stomachs and intestines. Stomach is a very sensitive organ and we must treat it with respect or it will boil and burn with anger, every time we irritate it. So avoid anything that angers your stomach. Also reduce *mental stress,* late night partying with less sleep; develop *regularity* in your habits and *e/ercise* moderately. Remember *green* is as good for your stomach as for the environment. Finally, lifestyle and diet modification should be the cornerstone of managing a case of hyperacidity, but where *infection* is a cause, certain antibiotics will help, and a short course of antacids will also do no harm; *but indiscriminate and prolonged acid suppression can sometimes lead to cancer. Also acid suppression drug called proton pump inhibitor (omeprazole)if used regularly can cause magnesium deficiency, leading to irregularity in heart beat, and osteoporosis. It can also lead to vitamin-B-12 and iron deficiency. Omeprazole also interferes with the action of Clopidogrel, a commonly used blood thinning drug. So, if you are taking medicines for acidity, take them under your doctor's supervision as far as possible.*

HYPERACIDITY & OESOPHAGIAL (GULLET) CANCER

Stomach has a protective layer of mucous, which protects it from excessive secretion of acid, but gullet has no such protection. If you suffer from heart burn or GERD (gastro esophageal reflux disease} which is due to stomach contents rising up into the gullet, the resulting effect of acid on the unprotected esophagus results in injury & pain. Repeated such attacks can lead to cancer, which is 45 times more common in these patients & is of a particularly aggressive kind.

HOW TO PREVENT HEARTBURN OR GERD

A ring like structure made of muscles, separates the gullet from the stomach and prevents the contents of the latter from regurgitating upwards into the former. If this structure, also called sphincter, becomes weak due to any cause it results in attacks of heartburn also called Gastro-esophageal-reflux disease or GERD. This can be prevented by the following measures-

1. Avoid foods like chocolate, peppermint, alcohol, onions, garlic, radish & fatty foods, which can relax the sphincter. Carbonated & caffeinated beverages can also do the same by causing bloating & acid overload in the stomach.

2. Avoid large meals

3. Fat accumulation in the abdomen can exert pressure on the stomach. So losing weight may help

4. Avoid tight belts & clothing.

5. Nicotine can relax the sphincter, so avoid smoking & intake of tobacco.

6. Never lie down & eat

7. If you suffer from nighttime attacks, elevate the head end of your bed with blocks.

8. In very severe cases, surgery to tighten the sphincter can be undertaken.

PEPTIC ULCER

If there is prolonged acidity, it can lead to erosion of the stomach and formation of an 'ulcer'. If this ulcer is in the stomach, it is called 'gastric ulcer', and if in the first part of the intestines after the stomach, it is called 'duodenal ulcer'. Most ulcers develop due to the causes of increased acid secretion listed above and due to an infection with a bacterium called 'H Pylori'. Aspirin and non steroidal anti inflammatory drugs like ibuprofen and naproxen can also cause them. Diagnosis of both an ulcer and H Pylori infection can be made by performing 'Gastroscopy' in which the stomach is visualized through a self illuminated flexible tube with a camera at the end, that is introduced into it, and a sample of contents also taken to examine for H Pylori infection. A breath test for detecting the bacterium can also be performed. Barium meal test is another alternative that helps in diagnosis.

Sometimes there can be complications like bleeding, perforation of the stomach, or narrowing of the affected part when the ulcer heals.

Management is with acid suppressant drugs, and drugs that form a protective barrier on the inner wall of the stomach called 'mucosal protective drugs' that help in healing of the ulcer. Other methods of treatment are lifestyle changes including diet and exercise, antibiotics to eradicate H Pylori infection, and if all else fails—surgery.

Surgery consists of cutting part of the 'vagus' nerve that stimulates acid secretion, or cutting off part of the stomach called 'antrum' that secretes a hormone which stimulates acid secretion.

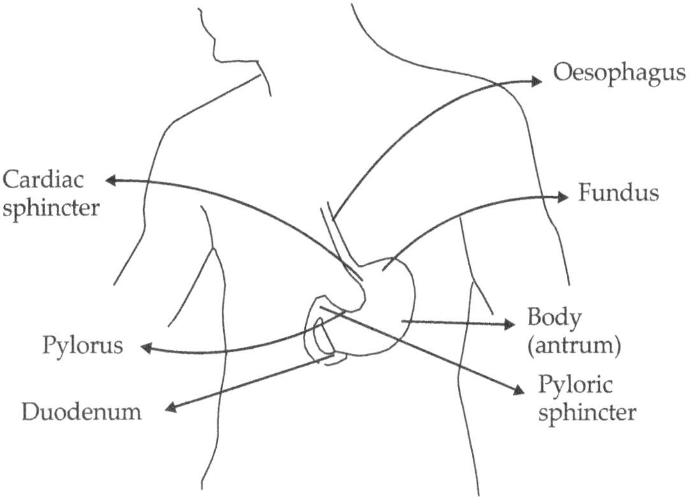

If there is narrowing of the stomach at its junction with the intestines called duodenum, it can be corrected by another surgical procedure called 'pyloroplasty'. All these surgeries can now be performed by laparoscopy involving very tiny incisions.

CASE STUDY

Mrs. X, a fifty- five-year-old obese lady suffered from backache and chronic fatigue and every possible test done on her for two years including X-rays, sonography and scans proved negative. She was told to stop her self-pity and to exercise, but she steadfastly maintained that she could not do so. Even psychiatric treatment did not help. Ultimately a special review consultation was conducted, and the patient revealed symptoms of hyperacidity so far considered unimportant by her and denied vehemently each time history was taken. She was put on a diet, and medication for hyperacidity, and both her backache and fatigue disappeared.

CASE STUDY

Mr. Y, a patient 60 years of age, presented with complaints of hyperacidity of a month's duration. Considering his age, he was subjected to investigations, which revealed advanced cancer of the stomach, which had spread all over the body, and he passed away in three months. So remember, sudden attacks of acidity in an older patient should always call for medical attention.

CASE STUDY

Mr-K, a 50 year old case of chronic mild hyperacidity, showing mild gastritis on gastroscopy, was tired of taking medicines and went for naturopathy treatment where he was administered two cups of salt and told his hyperacidity would be cured. Within a month, he developed severe pain in his stomach that did not respond to conventional treatment and he had to be admitted after he had a bout of haematemesis (blood vomiting). When he was stable, a gastroscopy was performed that he had a huge ulcer that was treated. But three months later he had to be re-admitted for repeated bouts of haematemesis and a repeat gastroscopy revealed a cancerous growth. Even after two surgeries, Mr. K passed away. The salt had eaten away his stomach lining and caused a rapidly growing cancer. So if you are looking for unconventional cures, go to a qualified person and not a quack. And it may be a good idea to talk to your regular doctor about the treatment modalities before going through with it.

APHTHOUS - ULCERS

These are ulcers in the mouth experienced by all of us some time or the other, and can be very painful and recurrent, in some patients. They may occur due to mental stress, hyperacidity, constipation, infections in mouth, sharp teeth, smoking tobacco and betel chewing, etc. So look out for these causes, but if they persist for too long remember they could be due to cancer, so don't ignore them. Besides medications a bland diet, and soothing applications like honey, glycerine, butter, coconut oil etc., can help in healing them.

INDIGESTION

'Gas' or 'dyspepsia' is very common after forty. Here the causes can be many -

1.   Constipation

2.   Hyperacidity

3.   Infections

4.   Diseases of liver

5.   Diseases of gall bladder

6.   Diseases of pancreas

7.   Certain medications

8.   Partial Intestinal obstruction

9.   Normal bloating due to increased fibre intake

10.   Any new indigestion may be due to *intestinal cancer*

The cause has to be found and treated along with yoga and exercise. Enzyme preparations should not be taken indiscriminately unless specifically indicated.

✦✦✦✦

2

Constipation

*"Training is every thing; the peach was once a bitter almond;
Cauliflower is nothing but cabbage with a college education".*
- Mark Twain

Bowels are an obsession with most of us. Every patient wants an early morning, single and total evacuation of his or her intestinal contents. Anything less than this ideal state leaves them dissatisfied. Remember, each of us is born with a certain kind of constitutional bowel habit but we can train it to act regularly to a great extent. But any amount of management can only modify but not totally change it unless harmful methods are used like strong cathartics or tobacco. What is normal bowel movement? - I'm afraid no one can answer this. Our physiology textbook cites two cases, - both of whom considered themselves normal, both extreme cases. One revealed he had seven privies (toilets) from his home to his office and visited all of them, and the other had no bowel movements from June of one year to May of the next year, and then complained of abdominal discomfort; the alarmed doctors, feeling all those lumps, opened him up and had the time of their lives cleaning out one year's accumulation! (Physiology textbooks don't lie!) Bawdy jokes abound about this serious problem. An educated man and a rustic were discussing how each of them woke up every morning. The city-bred spoke of the gentle song of the birds and snapping open of flowers as his morning alarm. The earthy rustic however had no use for such gentility and proclaimed that it was his bowels, that performed this useful function for him! Ancient Spartans were known to block their bowels before going to war. Apparently they came to no harm when they unblocked themselves later! I also remember one admitted patient on whom all our attempts to induce passage of stools failed for a fortnight. The relatives tried super human medication in the form of 'offerings' from a temple and it worked. The jubilant gentleman treated the whole ward to sweets!

Seriously, what can we do to ameliorate any severe constipation problem? First of all, as I mentioned earlier, minor problems should be left alone. For the more serious ones, diet and lifestyle changes and finally mild medication may be tried. Firstly, the problem has to be identified. Is it due to less bulk in the stools or due to reduced motility? If due to less bulk, we should reduce non-vegetarian intake (which leaves very little residue and therefore no bulk), take plenty of liquids, and food with a lot of soluble and insoluble fibre—skin, peel, core of fruits, vegetables, sprouts, salads, whole grains, beans, fenugreek, oats etc. Honey in water, prunes & a few drops of coconut oil in hot milk, are age-old remedies.

For reduced motility, exercise and yoga also definitely help, and acupressure and acupuncture may also be tried. If these measures do not work, mild laxatives and stool softeners like psyllium husk (isapgol) may be tried. Strong laxatives act as cathartics and wear off the lining of the intestines and should not be taken for long. Naturopathic treatment like enemas and mud packs are also said to help.

Finally, whatever methods are employed in treating

constipation, including over-the-counter drugs, make sure you discuss with your doctor regarding their long term safety, and don't go searching for utopia!

TOBACCO AND SMOKING

Tobacco is a cause of constipation, and apparently a help too. Many patients do not have bowel movements unless they chew tobacco or smoke a cigarette, but consuming tobacco continuously over a period of time leads to loss of bowel rugosity (muscle tone) and its contractile function, leading to permanent constipation, besides increasing the tendency towards oral and gastrointestinal cancer three fold!

MASS REFLEX

Early morning, on awakening, there is a movement of the whole bowel as one, which is called mass reflex. This reflex, leads to bowel evacuation, and should not be ignored or suppressed, or it will lead to chronic constipation.

Constipation accompanied by straining if left untreated can also lead to piles, fissure and prolapse of rectum (descent of end of intestines).

PILES

There are certain veins in our anal canal, which are called internal hemorrhoidal (deep inside anal canal) plexus, and external haemorrhoidal plexus (near the exterior). These haemorrhoidal plexii act as cushions to protect the anal sphincter from injury during stool passage. When they are subjected to continuous pressure as a result of hard stools or repeated straining during its passage, they become tortuous(twisted) and can burst, leading to burning, pain and bleeding after stools. This is what you understand as piles, also called hemorrhoids. Internal piles are normally painless unless they develop a blood clot and become thrombosed (blocked). Piles can also occur without constipation whenever there is increased pressure in the veins as in pregnancy and cirrhosis (a chronic liver disease).

Diagnosis

Even a visual examination may be enough to diagnose piles. For internal piles, one may need an anoscope or proctoscope --- (a hollow self lighted tube) to visualize it and also to rule out other causes of bleeding and pain from rectum.

Treatment

Increasing fiber intake to soften stools (dietary and simple natural fibers like psyllium husk (isapgol) plenty of water and certain medicines including ointments and creams, which reduce the problem, should treat it, and finally surgery if needed to cut and tie-up those blood vessels, that are severely involved. External piles can usually be managed without surgery but internal ones often do not respond without operation.

Other procedures

- ✦ Rubber band ligation—this is a procedure where elastic bands are applied around an internal haemorrhoid which then withers and falls off in a week's time. Performed correctly, the success rate is high.

- ✦ Sclerotherapy—involves injection of a liquid like phenol into the haemorrhoid which then shrivels up.

- ✦ Electric cauterisation(burning) of the piles

- ✦ Laser treatment

- ✦ Cryo (freezing) treatment

- ✦ Infra-red radiation Surgery

- ✦ Surgical excision of the hemorrhoids

- ✦ Doppler (sonography) assisted tying up of the hemorrhoids

- ✦ Stapling procedure

If the anal sphincter that controls stool passage becomes very tight, it traps a prolapsed haemorrhoid outside the anus—this is called strangulation.

George Brett a base ball player left a game in 1980 due to haemorrhoidal pain and when he came back after surgery and getting cured, he famously said - 'my problems are all behind me'!

FISSURE, ULCER AND FISTULA

Due to hard stools there may be an erosion or tear of the superficial layer of the anal canal, which is called fissure. Sometimes they become deep and chronic and are called anal ulcers. A healed ulcer can lead to contracture or narrowing of the anal passage. Fistula is a tract leading from the external opening of anus to the rectum and is formed due to healing of anal abscesses (pus filled pockets). Fissures can be very painful, and typically the person is so uncomfortable that he will not be able to even sit on a chair. I think that is why an obnoxious person is called a pain in the ass!

In adults, fissures may be caused by constipation, the passing of large, hard stools, or by prolonged diarrhea as well as anal sex. In older adults, anal fissures may be caused by decreased blood flow to the area. They also occur after child birth. Superficial fissures heal without treatment, but deep ones develop an ulcer and get infected leading to non –healing and require medical and even surgical help.

Non-surgical treatments

Non surgical treatment consists of stool softeners, local ointments containing drugs called nitroglycerine, calcium channel blockers (nifedipine and diltiazem), and injection of botulinum toxin locally to relax the sphincter and reduce pain.

Sitz bath

It is a very old form of treatment where the hips and buttocks are soaked in water with salt. Water can be hot, cold or alternating hot and cold. Hot Sitz baths are for haemorrhoids, muscle pains, painful genitals and ovaries, uterine cramps and prostatic pain. Cold Sitz baths help particularly in vaginal discharge and constipation. Alternating cold and hot Sitz baths help in abdominal colic, infections, and muscle and nerve pains. They also help to relieve swelling and water retention in body especially if salt is added to water.

Procedure

To prepare a Sitz bath, fill a tub or basin so that the water covers the hips and reaches the middle of the abdomen. When using a hot sitz bath, the bathtub or basin should be filled with water of about 110°F. Stay in the bath for twenty minutes. When using a cold sitz bath, fill the bathtub or basin with ice water. Stay in the cold bath for half a minute only.

When using alternating hot and cold baths, fill one basin with water of about 110°F, and a second basin with ice water. Immerse yourself first in the hot sitz bath, and remain there for three to four minutes. Then move to the cold sitz bath, and remain there for half a minute. Repeat this two to four times, and towel yourself dry.

Do check with your doctor whether there are any contraindications before taking sitz baths. Surgery for fissure Surgery is called 'Lateral sphincterotomy' and is a procedure where a tiny cut is made under general anaesthesia in the anal sphincter (the muscular ring that controls stool outflow) which has become tight. It also improves blood supply and promotes healing. The patient improves very fast but in some cases there can be a complication of stool incontinence (involuntary or uncontrolled stool passage).

Anal dilatation or stretching—in this procedure, the sphincter is not cut but dilated. Faecal (stool) incontinence (leaking) is commoner in this procedure. But a slower and more gradual method of dilatation done repeatedly in a graded fashion avoids side effects.

ANAL SKIN TAGS

These are small shapeless flaps that develop just outside the anal opening. They are also called 'achrocordons'. They occur in many anal problems like fissures and haemorrhoids. For example if a large haemorrhoid prolapsed outside heals, it leaves behind a 'tag'. Or they can occur after any surgery near the anus, or due to the irritation caused by tight underwear or if the area is not washed properly after passing stools. If they do not lead to any problems, they should be left alone. If there is pain or itching, they can be removed under local anaesthesia. When large in size or many in number, they will have to be removed under general anaesthesia. Laser surgery can also be performed.

RECTAL PROLAPSE

Constipation accompanied by straining if left untreated can also lead to prolapse of rectum (descent of end of intestines outside anus). It may have to be surgically repaired.

✦✦✦✦

3

Diarrhoea

The other side of the coin shows patients who are prone to diarrhoea. In some, it is transitory, and caused by irritant foods or mental stress. These cases normally respond to a simple anti–spasmodic drug and diet control. Diarrhoea may also be due to worms or infections, which can be diagnosed by three consecutive stool examinations, and treated accordingly. There is a condition called irritable bowel syndrome (IBS), which does not respond to routine medications, and needs drugs to reduce mental stress, and other supportive measures over a long period to ameliorate the condition.

After forty, we must also be aware that any persistent diarrhoea may be due to cancer, especially if there is blood in the stools.

DIET

Diet for diarrhoea, should be soft and easily digestible. Buttermilk (diluted yoghurt), green- ripe- bananas, gruels made of arrowroot, rice etc., black tea (absorbs gas and acts as binding agent), and isapgol or psyllium husk (helps in both constipation and diarrhoea) and plenty of well-diluted lemon juice with sugar and salt to replace salts and water lost in stools. If there is accompanying vomiting, a pinch of soda bicarbonate may also be added. Dry ginger powder quarter teaspoonful, with some jaggery (unrefined sugar), turmeric in buttermilk, carrot juice and half a teaspoonful of fenugreek seeds (methi) in water taken three times a day, also help in diarrhoea. Avoid milk, and spicy foods and foods that are difficult to digest.

A word of caution – do not take inadequate doses of self-prescribed anti diarrhoeals, as you may end up becoming a chronic purger, very difficult to cure.

Prevention of infective diarrhoeas is by avoiding taking anything uncooked and cold, outside the home like water, salads, chutneys, juices, unpackaged ice creams etc. At home too, fruits and salad vegetables should be thoroughly washed and scraped and subjected to a final soaking in water, to which a pinch of potassium permanganate can be added, to dislodge sticky dirt and wors.

CASE STUDY

Mrs. X, age forty years, presented with diarrhoea mixed with mucous and blood of fifteen years duration. At 5'2", she weighed thirty-six kilograms, and her hemoglobin was only six grams%. All possible investigations had already been done and were found to be negative.

She was put on a soft diet (boiled vegetables, mashed rice, no milk, rice and arrowroot gruels, strictly told to avoid taking anything outside the house and to drink only boiled water. She was also put on yeast powder, and Lactobacilli enriched curds (these are natural bacteria normally present in our intestines and fight infection), and soluble isapgol or psyllium husk (which is soluble fibre and helps both in diarrhoea and constipation.) Some supportive drugs were also used to reduce stress, which were gradually withdrawn over a period of six months. At the end of this period, she weighed sixty kilograms, her haemoglobin was thirteen grams%, and she was completely free of her problem. She was told to continue with boiled water and avoid eating out for another two years. It is now six years and with every visit, her blooming cheeks tell their own happy story! This is a classic case of diet, attitudinal change, and supportive medication working in tandem to bring about a cure.

IRRITABLE BOWEL SYNDROME (IBS)

Irritable bowel syndrome or irritable colon syndrome or spastic colon, is the most common gastrointestinal disease. It is twice as common in women than in men and usually occurs in the age group 18-40. It is of three types:

+ Spastic type—Presents with chronic abdominal pain and constipation.

+ Chronic intermittent diarrhoea without pain.

+ Alternating constipation and diarrhoea.

Why does it occur?

Intestines are like a long and twisted tube that is lined with muscles. These muscles *contract* to cause squeezing action that helps to push the contents forward. This squeezing action is normally supposed to occur only when bowel contents need to be pushed forwards. But if *resting motility of the colon* becomes excessive, or erratic (sometimes less sometimes more), it leads to IBS.

Mental stress very often acts like a trigger.

What are the complaints in IBS?

Complaints in IBS may be chronic constipation, diarrhoea, or both, for months or years, worse in morning, or after breakfast. Typically, there are three to four loose stools with mucous in the morning, the rest of the day being uneventful. There may be pasty, pencil like stools, with mucous, or just watery stools, *blood in stools is not seen in IBS*; so if you see blood, consult your doctor immediately. Abdominal cramps, pain and bloating are usually present which is relieved on passage of stools. Sometimes there is backache, weakness and even a feeling of faintness. The complaints may last for a few months and get cleared, or may remain permanently. Rarely pain can be so severe that it may interfere with routine activities.

Diagnosis

Diagnosis can be made by the long standing, and intermittent nature of the complaints, the fact that it does not affect physical well being to a great extent, and also on the basis of examination findings both physical and investigations, which will be normal.

Management of IBS

Remember, IBS can be alleviated but not totally cured. Patients should be made to understand this and encouraged to *adapt* themselves to the disease Pain reduction can often be achieved by a simple measure like a hot water bottle applied to the abdomen.

Cutting Alcohol and Tobacco

Irritable Bowel Syndrome is not a serious disease although it is very bothersome. You must learn to recognize the *triggers* that bring about the attack and try to avoid them. If you are a smoker, try to stop smoking or at least cut down. Oral tobacco chewing should similarly be stopped or reduced. Alcohol intake can also trigger off an attack, and if this is so, it should be avoided.

Exercise in IBS

Exercise is important as a sound body helps us to tolerate minor problems better, and reduces the severity of major ones.

Diet

Changing eating habits helps to a great extent in a patient of IBS. In some, the problem may be due to deficiency of an enzyme (enzymes are agents that facilitate chemical reactions in the body) called lactase that helps in digestion of milk and withdrawing milk products may help these patients. A soft diet that is easily digestible is best. Caffeine containing drinks like coffee, chocolates and colas should be avoided. Similarly many drinks contain sorbitol as artificial sweetener, which can trigger off an attack. Foods that are difficult to digest like whole pulses, whole legumes (rajma, kabuli chana), beans, should also be avoided as they may also precipitate an attack, especially in patients who have 'bloating' and intermittent diarrhea along with constipation. High carbohydrate and high fat foods should also be avoided. Soya products may be useful in IBS, like Tofu and Soya milk. Fluid intake should be increased and a high fiber diet stressed on. Ideally small frequent four-hourly meals should be consumed while trying to avoid overloading of stomach. A high fibre diet is beneficial in most patients especially where constipation is predominant. On the other hand, in those patients in whom 'gas' or 'bloating' is common, a high fibre diet may *add* to the problem.

Psychotherapy

Stress can act as a trigger for IBS; hence psychotherapy pays maximum dividends in its management. Almost 60% of patients show some improvement.

✦✦✦✦

4

Dental Care

As important as our eyes are our teeth and only those who don't have them can appreciate their importance. Besides gentle brushing of the teeth two to three times a day with up and down strokes, massage the gums with fingers and scrape the tongue gently but thoroughly Take good care of your gums because they are like cement and keep the teeth firmly in place. Biting and chewing food thoroughly not only strengthens gums and teeth ("If you don't use them, you will lose them!"), but also begins the process of digestion, since chewing stimulates saliva secretion which aids in digestion besides sending the food in a more easy to digest state into the stomach. Avoid tobacco, refined foods and sweets to keep the teeth healthy and eat enough greens and milk products to provide calcium and vitamins, which are needed to keep your teeth strong.

Acidity can wear off gums and enamel (covering of tooth), and thus weaken our dentures, so if you suffer from gastric reflux disease (acid coming up into the mouth), get it attended to. Chronic infections, vitamin C deficiency, thyroid hypo- function, (reduced functioning) and certain epilepsy and blood pressure medicines can also weaken our gums. Remember a good set of teeth not only keep us looking young but also keep the body healthy.

Upper teeth should be brushed above downward and lower ones below upwards. Eat a carrot, apple or cucumber after meals to cleanse the teeth thoroughly.

Common dental problems seen after forty are: -

1. Food sticking between or inside teeth
2. Bleeding from gums or gaps in teeth
3. Loose or shaky teeth
4. Increase in gaps between teeth
5. Growing out or shifting of teeth
6. Cracks in teeth
7. Sensitivity of teeth to cold, hot or sour food
8. Chipping off of tooth
9. Dull pain in jaw or face
10. A sharp edge to some teeth
11. Burning sensation in teeth on eating spicy food
12. Difficulty in eating from one side although there is no pain

Around forty, it is a good idea to have a thorough dental check-up along with other tests, to make sure there are no problems, which need immediate attention, otherwise visit your dentist when you have any of the problems outlined above.

Now let us understand a few common dental procedures:

DISCOLOURED TEETH

Discolouration of teeth may be due to--

+ Coffee, Tea, Colas
+ Antibiotics in children
+ Accidents-after accidental chipping of tooth it loses its whiteness

✦ After root canal treatment also teeth get discoloured

Management of discoloured teeth---is by bleaching, applying a veneer layer, or by covering it with a white'cap'.

HYPERSENSITIVE TEETH

Teeth become hypersensitive when the nerves inside the dentin get exposed due to wearing off of the enamel (see picture below) It can range from a mild irritation to an intense shooting pain. This typically increases when the teeth get exposed to something too cold or hot, sweet, sour, or sudden pressure.

Treatment is in the form of some chemicals like amorphous calcium and phosphate, , potassium nitrate, strontium chloride, fluoride therapy, or calcium sodium phosphosilicate to coat the teeth. But the response is only partial.

Cut Section of One Tooth

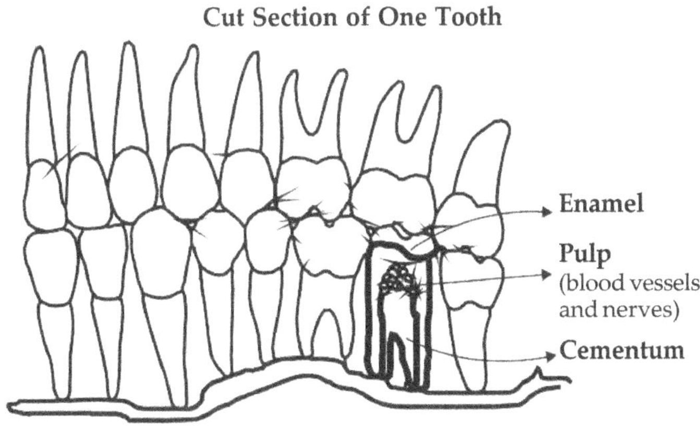

The mode of action is linked to their ability to form mineralised deposits within the tubule lumen and on the surface of the exposed dentine that prevents direct contact with the nerves.

These chemicals are available for home use in desensitizing toothpastes or dentifrices, potassium salts, mouthwashes and chewing gums for home use. Gastro-esophageal reflux disease (GERD) –where acid from the stomach regurgitates into the mouth, is another common cause of sensitive teeth since the acid wears off the enamel. Treatment is for acidity — discussed in the first chapter.

Treatment at the Dentist's Office

This may include the application of dental sealants, having fillings put over the exposed root that is causing the sensitivity, or a recommendation to wear a specially made night guard where the cause is GERD or teeth grinding at night. All the chemicals available for home use can also be used for application under pressure using special instruments. Laser treatment is also used.

Prevention

Prevention is by avoiding all abrasive irritants and acidity causing foods that lead to wearing off of the enamel.

TOOTH DECAY

Tooth decay, is caused by interaction between bacteria and food particles in the mouth. Debris (waste matter) collects in the crevices between teeth. This is called **a** plaque, and usually it is invisible. Living bacteria inside the plaques ferment foods producing acid. This acid now dissolves enamel, allowing bacteria to invade the inner structures, and slowly the tooth is destroyed. Infection can also enter the tooth directly through break in the enamel.

PERIODONTAL DISEASE

Here the problem starts below the gum, leading to plaque formation and later it hardens to form what is called 'tartar'. Little pockets are formed in the gum, where bacteria collect, and slowly the tooth gets loosened from the jaw.

GUM DISEASE

Bleeding gums show that a break has occurred at the gum line. It can be due to infection, scurvy (deficiency of vitamin-C), some bleeding disorders, some drugs that cause gingivitis (inflamed gums) like blood pressure lowering medicines called calcium channel blockers, anti cancer drug called cyclosporine, anti epilepsy drug called phenytoin, and drugs that cause bleeding from any part of the body like aspirin.

ROOT CANAL TREATMENT

Root is the part of the tooth, embedded into the jaw. Internally the tooth has a *pulp cavity* at the crown and *root canal* at the base. It is in the root canal, that infection collects and may have to be drilled and removed since it cannot repair itself like the rest of the tissues in the body. It is then 'filled' with material so that it does not collect again. This is called root canal treatment.

Silver fillings are not so popular nowadays, as they leak, can get oxidized and blacken, also lead to allergic reactions.

Newer filling materials are modified bio compatible plastics which are variously graded as - composite, compomer, ceromer and ormosers, the last of which is the latest. These impart a natural colour, and some of them are fluoride or silica fortified to maintain strength, making them superior to the older ones but remember there is no such thing as a permanent filling. After the treatment the tooth can be 'capped' for better cosmetic results.

OTHER ADVANCES IN DENTISTRY

1. Bone grafting for any loss of bone especially after cancer surgery.

2. Aero- rotors with coolant water for painless drilling.

3. Newer Dentures - All of you would like to know about dentures. These may be partial or total and again removable or fixed. All dentures nowadays are made of poly-methyl – methacryalate.

Partial – dentures can be made for one or two missing teeth and fixed using normal teeth as a bridge. They are made of nickel chrome or beryllium chrome and covered with ceramic.

Total dentures can be removable or fixed.

+ Removable dentures are the ones commonly used. The cost can vary according to the amount of material, type of material, number of sittings needed to achieve perfection etc.

+ Fixed Dentures - Here holes are drilled in the jaws, some screws put in, and regular dentures fixed on to them. Eight screws are needed; four for each jaw and these teeth are now permanently fixed like natural teeth, giving better cosmetic effect and utility. Since they are fixed to the jaw, brushing and cleaning them is also easier. The only problem is of chances of resorption (wearing off) of the bone surrounding the screws, leading to problems later. The perfect denture is therefore yet to be developed, a denture tailored to a person's mouth and face.

SOME ORAL EXERCISES:

Here are a few useful exercises, which can be performed after brushing the teeth, which not only strengthen them but also tone up all the systems of our body.

1   Using your thumb and your index finger, massage the gums of the upper jaw, pulling downward. Similarly massage the gums of the lower jaw and pull them upwards.

    Benefit : This exercise increases the blood circulation around your gums, teeth and their roots.

2   Using sliding movements of the forefingers of both hands, massage from the centre of the forehead to the temple.

    Benefit : The circulation of blood improves in the head and you feel fresh.

3   Stretch your tongue out, and using the thumb and the index fingers of both the hands, pull the tongue out as though milking a cow.

    Benefit : The thyroid and the parathyroid glands, which play an important role in body metabolism, get stimulated.

4   Place the first three fingers of your right hand at the root of the tongue and tickle there. You may feel like vomiting.

    Benefit : The stored phlegm is cleared and thrown out.

5   Take a mouthful of water, hold your breath and start splashing water over your face. This creates negative pressure and helps loosen up the congestion of the mucous lining in the nose. Spit out the water and blow out your nose, closing one nostril.

    Benefit : This is good for sinusitis. The splashing of the water will also enhance the glow of your facial skin, ward off dark circles, and keep the skin smooth and wrinkle-free.

Finally, remember no one can replicate what nature has given us whether it is our brain or our dentures, so take care of your precious pearls and **KEEP SMILING!**

✦✦✦✦

5

Windows of Body and Soul
EYES

Bright, alert and clear eyes tell us that all is well with the body and mind. On the other hand dull, droopy, dry, smudgy, or blood shot eyes tell their own story. They are the windows of not only the soul but the body too, and aid in maintaining balance and equilibrium.

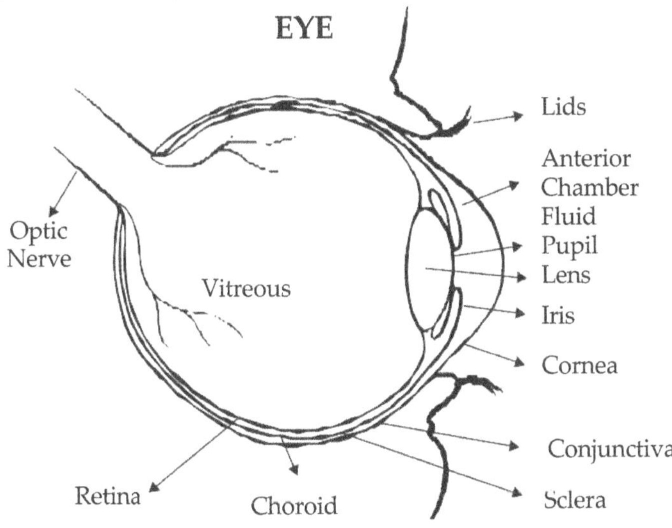

Any change in the eyes including visual defects (sudden or gradual), discolouration, floating spots etc. should be immediately brought to the notice of your doctor. Human eye is like a camera where the light filters in through the cornea, and lens and forms an inverted image on the retina. This image is then carried by the optic nerve to the brain and "printed' after straightening it, and visualized by us as a picture.

Light enters through the pupil, which adjusts in size according to its brightness. In sunlight, pupil is almost like a pinpoint and at night it is dilated (becomes big). After passing through the pupils, light enters the lens, which adjusts itself to receive it. From there it is focused on to the retina. When light is in colour or focused vision is required as for reading, it strikes the 'fovea' that carries cones but otherwise it strikes the rods. The light bleaches these rods, and the resulting chemical process triggers off a tiny wave of electricity. This current now stimulates the optic nerve behind the retina, which swiftly carries the message to the 'optic centre' in the brain. The brain interprets the image as say a snake and orders – 'withdraw!' All this takes 1/200th of a second!

Eyes rest by working in tandem – while one eye rests by working only 10% of its capacity, the other eye carries the burden by working 90%. They keep doing this in turns. We only have two eyes, and overworking them can lead to complications. In contrast, a butterfly has 12000 eyes, so each of its eyes must be getting plenty of rest!

Our eyes were not designed for so much near work. Stone Age man needed mainly distant vision to hunt his food. But as mankind evolved, he has to do more of 'near vision' work. Eyes have not evolved enough to cope with this load, leading to problems like myopia (short sightedness) and hypermetropia (long sightedness). With most of us working at computers these problems are only going to multiply! This is also why we see so many youngsters wearing glasses.

CARE OF EYES:

Taking care of your eyes should be part of your daily routine. Splashing cold water two to three times a day cleanses and stimulates the eyes, as does looking at the early morning rising sun through interlaced fingers. Reading, working with the computer or watching T.V. for long hours, puts a lot of strain on the eyes, which can be avoided by distance viewing for a few seconds every 30 minutes or so and frequent blinking.

'Palming' is a very relaxing exercise for tired eyes. Here the interlaced fingers of the hands are used to cover the open eyes such that no light can enter, and then an attempt is made to visualise total blackness. When that happens, the eyes automatically feel rested. Other useful exercises are 'swinging' the eyes from side to side, alternate distance and near fixation, and reading Snellen's chart (the chart used by eye doctors) with one eye at a time, the chart being fixed at six meters distance. U.V. filter glasses, protect the eyes from the harmful rays emanating from computers, & recently there has been a study where quartz has been reported to absorb these rays.

NUTRITION FOR EYES:

Milk and its products, greens, yellow fruits and vegetables, fish and almonds are good for the eyes. Incidentally fish and almonds are shaped like eyes - coincidence? Or is nature telling us something?

Now let us consider some common eye problems after forty –

PRESBYOPIA:

The commonest eye problem after forty is presbyopia, due to hardening of lens and laxity of its supporting muscles, leading to receding of near vision and corrected by glasses for doing near work, like reading.

RED EYE

Red eyes are a common problem and can be due to various causes, but they should never be taken lightly since sometimes the cause may be a serious one. It is always advisable to consult a doctor and treat the cause which can be -

+ Irritation due to a foreign body--a speck of dust or any other foreign body may enter the eye and cause irritation, leading to a red eye. Blink frequently without rubbing to try and dislodge the foreign body and if it fails, see an eye-doctor.

+ Contact lenses--in many people, wearing contact lenses for an extended period of time can cause redness of the eyes. This may be due to allergy or dryness. Try using moisturizing eye drops but if it fails, see your doctor.

+ Injury to eye-- direct injury to the eye due to any cause will lead to redness, and any blunt injury around the eyes, including head injury will also lead to redness and later a black eye. Immediately apply ice and see your doctor.

+ Conjunctivitis -a common cause is conjunctivitis that is inflammation of the outer protective layer of the eye. It can be due to allergies, or infections. Most attacks are self limiting and get all right on their own, but if severe and persistent, see your doctor.

+ Uveitis and blepharitis - infection in the 'uvea' or eyelids(blephara) can also cause redness - consult an ophthalmologist.

+ Dry eyes - long standing dryness of the eyes can cause the blood vessels to dilate in an attempt to moisturize the eyes, leading to redness - use moisturizing drops.

+ Ulcer or infection in the cornea- cornea is the cover of the central dome-like part of the eye, and when it gets infected, the surrounding blood vessels become prominent, leading to a red eye - consult an ophthalmologist.

+ A burst blood vessel - sometimes a blood vessel can burst leading to bleeding - it may be due to a hard sneeze, cough, severe bout of vomiting, high blood pressure or some bleeding disorders - apply ice and see your doctor.

+ Acute angle glaucoma - in this condition, there is sudden blockage in the flow of fluid from one chamber of the eye to the other (explained below under 'glaucoma'), leading to severe pain accompanied by redness. In most cases it is an emergency and if not treated immediately, it can lead to blindness - consult ophthalmologist.

STYE

Stye is also called 'hardeolum' and is an infection in the sebaceous (oil secreting) glands in the eyelids. They are small yellowish red nodules that are quite painful but get all right in a week. If they persist, or recur frequently, diabetes should be suspected. Hot fomentation is the home remedy of choice. Pain killers, local ointments and oral antibiotics may be prescribed by your doctor. As a last resort, surgery may be needed in a few cases. If the 'meibomian sebaceous glands on the inside of the lids are affected, it is called'chalazion'. *Chalazions* are normally painless but do not get all right fast. Chalazions frequently need surgical intervention.

DRY EYES

Eyes are kept lubricated and moist by means of tears that contain secretions from various glands. Tears contain water, oils, mucus, and lysozymes (antibacterial). When secretion from any or all the glands is reduced, there is dryness.

Symptoms - there may be a gritty sensation, sensitivity to light, mild pain, itching or redness.

Causes

+ Old age

+ After menopause in women

+ Thyroid deficiency

+ Working in an Air conditioned or heated environment

+ Medicines like diuretics, anti histaminics and contraceptive pills

+ Diseases like Rheumatoid arthritis and Sjogren's syndrome

+ Any defect in the eyes that prevent them from shutting or blinking.

Treatment

Artificial tears are available as eye drops that will keep the eyes moist. The tear duct that drains off tears into the nose can be blocked so that whatever tears are secreted, will remain in the eyes.

GLAUCOMA:

It is increase in the fluid pressure inside the eyes. Normal pressure is less than 20 mm of mercury. Certain eye drops and oral medicines can reduce the pressure, but if they do not work, surgery has to be resorted to relieve it.

Glaucoma can be open angle or closed angle. In closed angle glaucoma, the angle from which the fluid drains out is suddenly blocked, leading to rapid rise in pressure in the eyes and is accompanied by severe headache, which makes him rush to the doctor, but open angle glaucoma is slowly progressive and the patient may think he is suffering from cataract and ignore the problem, leading to blindness.

DIABETES AND HYPERTENSION:

Hypertension and diabetes affect the blood vessels on the retina (the screen behind the eyes). If too many of these vessels get affected and bleeding occurs, it is dangerous. *Laser* can be used to stop the bleeding by sealing the blood vessels.

MACULAR DEGENERATION OF OLD AGE

Here there is a gradual loss of central vision and laser treatment can help, or a special lens can be fitted after removing the existing one.

CATARACT SURGERY:

Gone are the days when the eye was cut open, lens removed, and thick heavy glasses given to substitute them.

Newer Methods:

1. **Intra ocular lens implant** - In this procedure, the lens is removed, and an artificial one introduced inside, thus avoiding the need to wear thick glasses.

2. **Phaco emulsification** - Here a very small 3 mm cut is made in the cornea (outermost layer of eye), an ultrasonic probe

introduced, the lens broken up into pieces by sonic rays and the pieces sucked out. Later a foldable lens is introduced. Healing is fast and restoration of vision almost immediate. Sometimes the bag holding the intraocular lens becomes opaque and it has to be removed by laser, which can be done without admitting the patient.

RETINAL DEGENERATION

This is weakening of retina, and either *c r y o* (gas at sub zero temperature) or laser is used to fuse it to the second layer of the eye called choroid, thus preventing the retina from getting 'detached' and causing blindness.

EYE DONATION

In many young people, due to infection, the outermost layer of eyes called cornea becomes opaque and the person cannot see. If you pledge your eyes after death, two people may get restoration of vision. So gift your eyes. You need to understand that the whole eyeball is not removed, and any eye doctor can be called who will remove only the superficial outer layer. It should be done within six to eight hours of death. Eyes should be immediately closed after the patient dies and if possible, antibiotic drops instilled, to make sure the eyes remain infection-free & moist for donation.

✦ ✦ ✦ ✦

6

Ears

"Give every man thy ear but few thy voice"

This is a good axiom to follow, as it keeps us out of mischief, and we utilise more of these beautiful pieces of architecture called – ears.

EAR

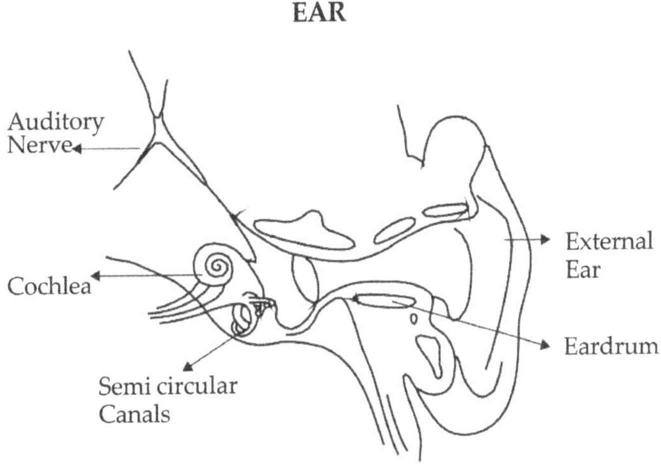

HOW WE HEAR

Consider a trumpet, divided into 3 parts - outer part receives the sound waves and transmits it on to a stretched membrane (like the top of a drum – hence called ear drum); this in turn vibrates at the same frequency as the sound waves received, and transmits it onto three little bones in the middle ear called 'Malleus' shaped like a hammer, 'Incus' (shaped like the anvil of a cobbler,) and 'Stapes' (shaped like the stirrup on a horse- (where the horse rider places his feet when he climbs on to the horse). These tiny bones not only transmit sound, they amplify it 20 fold before passing it on to the inner ear to an organ called the cochlea. The main organ of hearing is the cochlea, a snail like structure whose coils are filled with thousands of hairs, each of which is tuned to recognise a particular type of sound wave.

These hairs now wave about in the fluid in the same frequency they have received, producing a miniscule amount of electricity that is transmitted to the auditory nerve that conducts the message to the hearing centre in the brain. The brain now deciphers the code it has received and we come to know what we have heard. Some amount of sound is also conducted directly through the bones of the face into the ear.

The whole process is so fast that there does not seem any latent period, between the sound created by a source and its recognition by us. Imagine the amazing amount of automation which has gone into this whole process of hearing, which we tend to take so much for granted. Human body has enough neural networking and computing equal to many super computers put together. In fact each organ in the body is so complex that we may never be able to replicate them however hard we try. Also we need to understand that every cell, tissue and organ is connected in some way to all the others in the body and it is near impossible to figure out all these inter connections.

A baby can discern sound waves vibrating at frequencies between 16 - 30 K hertz per second. Gradually the upper limit of hearing drops till at 80 we may hear only about not more than 4 K hertz/sec. *Decibel* is a measure of intensity of sound. Animals can hear much higher frequencies of sound.

MAINTAINING BALANCE

The inner ear also performs the function of maintaining balance besides that of hearing. Nature considers the inner ear so important that it is enclosed by the hardest bone in the body and filled with fluid to provide additional protection. There are three 'semi circular' loops or canals besides the cochlea in the inner ear, along with fluid which has some floating particles called 'otoliths' These semicircular canals, are sensitive to any change in position of the body. One is directed so that it detects up and down movement of body, the other sideways movement and a 3rd forward and backward movement. Normally when the body moves in any one direction, these fluid canals bend with the movement and convey this information to the brain. The brain now orders the opposing muscles of the body to contract so that the person does not take a sudden fall. If the movements are too fast, as in a turbulent ship, a fast and lurching bus or on a roller coaster ride, the canals may get confused, and unable to convey the change in body position quickly enough to the brain leading to severe giddiness and sometimes a feeling of nausea, sweating, and even vomiting. Many of us suffer from this motion sickness and are thus not able to travel in a bus for a long distance ride. There are tablets available to prevent this from happening. Certain drugs and infections can also cause giddiness, 'ringing' sounds in the ears, and even deafness. Once the problem occurs, it may take a few days, weeks or months to settle down. Medication, if taken, should not be continued beyond six weeks, as it may interfere with the body's ability to acclimatize.

Middle ear is connected to the throat by a tube called *Eustachian tube*. That is why any infection in the throat can be transmitted to the ear and vice versa.

WAX

Ear secretes an oily substance to trap dust particles which enter it, and throws it out in the form of 'wax'. There is a self-expelling mechanism for this, so there is no need to poke and clean your ears (you might push the wax further in, and 'impact' it). After a bath, put a finger into the ear through a thin towel, shake it thoroughly and then clean. This is sufficient to dislodge and remove any extra wax. If there is hardening of any accumulated wax, instill wax-softening drops daily for a week. It will facilitate expulsion, but in severe cases, it is better to consult an ENT specialist.

EAR DISCHARGE

Discharge from the ears should always be taken seriously, otherwise permanent deafness and worse, even infection to the brain can ensue. Those who are prone to ear discharge should protect their ears with cotton plugs while bathing, going out in a fast moving vehicle or when it is very cold.

DEAFNESS

Certain types of deafness can be cured, where the cause is a damaged cochlea. Cochlea as already explained is a snail like structure in the ear, which acts as a receiver for the sound waves and transmits it to the auditory nerve, which in turn conveys the message to the brain for deciphering. Artificial cochlear implants have been created which after implanting in the ear behave like the healthy cochlea, thus leading to restoration of hearing. The only problem is the cost, which can be prohibitive.

SOUND POLLUTION

We are constantly being made aware of air pollution, but an equally serious problem is that of sound pollution which is largely ignored

Continuous exposure to high intensity sound over a period of time or very high intensity sound even once can damage our cochlea leading to hearing loss. Anything more than 85 decibels of sound is harmful for the ears. Now consider the following noise levels -

Jet take off (can cause permanent hearing loss)	-	150	decibels
Rock concert	-	120	decibels
Steel mill	-	110	decibels
Loudspeaker	-	100 – 120	decibels!
Noisy Street	-	90	decibels!

Recommended WHO guidelines -

A) Residential areas	-	6am-9pm	55db
		9pm-6am	45db
B) Silent zones	-	6am-9pm	50db
		9pm-6am	40db

Ill effects of noise

Noise can affect us in many ways. Some of these are-

1)   Interference in communication

2)   Disturbance in sleep

3)   Stress related diseases, especially hypertension, migraine & mental problems

4)   Interference with one's occupation

5)   Invasion of privacy

6)   Disruption of social interaction

7)   Accidents

8)   Temporary hearing loss

9)   Permanent hearing loss

So whenever possible, (unless you are driving) protect your ears from loud sound.

The rate and intensity at which we are being exposed to noise, very soon we may be needing hearing aids, so let us understand something about them!

HEARING AIDS

Hearing aids can be   -

+ Behind the ear model,

+ Partially in the ear

+ Completely in ear canal

+ Eye glass model

As a rule the smaller the hearing aid the lesser the power, except for the latest generation fully digital models, which are small but also powerful.

How they work:

Hearing aids amplify sounds from our surroundings and convey them to the auditory (hearing nerve). Normally this is the work of the cochlea. The sounds are carried by the nerve to the hearing center in the brain, for deciphering and making sense of what has been conveyed to it, using its memory bank.

Acclimatization

It may take a month *to get used to* your hearing aid. Start with a quiet place and then only move on to busy streets slowly; otherwise you might get frustrated with the inability to filter out extraneous sounds. When choosing a hearing aid, it is better to opt for a tested and trusted brand, with a warranty.

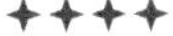

7

Nose

Grecian, flat, or Mongoloid, whatever the shape,
nose is a very useful part of the body.

NOSE AND SINUSES

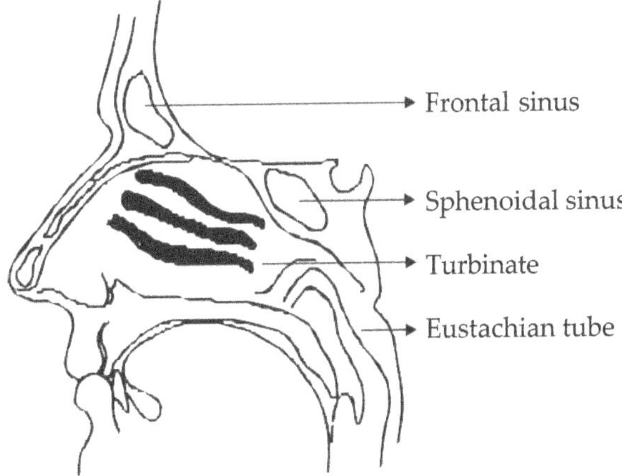

Nose lies between the roof of the mouth, eyes and the brain and is divided internally by a 'septum' or partition into two equal parts called nostrils. It is also connected to small hollows in the facial bone called *sinuses*. In the cheeks there are the *ma/illary sinuses*, above the eyes and in the forehead are the *frontal sinuses,*

between nose and eyes in front are the *ethmoid sinuses*, and there are two sinuses behind, called the *Sphenoid sinuses.* These hollow spaces were created by nature to make the skull lighter so that our delicate neck could support it. But wherever there is space it tends to get occupied and in the case of sinuses, it gets occupied by mucous that clogs them whenever there is an infection or allergic reaction—a condition we call 'sinusitis'.

Nose, is responsible for four important functions –conditioning of air, filtration of air, fighting infections, and sense of smell.

CONDITIONING OF AIR

The air we breathe is either too warm or too cold. Nose is provided with a network of tiny blood vessels near its entrance called 'Littles' area'. These blood vessels expand whenever the body gets warmed up, so that more heat can be lost to the outside. On the other hand, when it is cold, these blood vessels contract to reduce heat loss from the body. Warming the air is also a function of 'turbinates'. These are little chips of bone that can be felt on the sidewalls of the nostrils. If the air is very cold, these turbinates swell up and increase their surface area of blood vessels thus warming the air that enters through the nose.

FILTRATION AND CLEANING

Filtration and cleaning is performed by small hairs and by secretion of mucous, about a litre of which is secreted a day. This mucous traps dirt and ensures that clean air enters the lungs. What is surprising is that we don't realize the amount of fluid being secreted inside such a small space. This is because, it is secreted a little at a time to provide continuous cleaning throughout the day, as we breathe in and breathe out. Mucous acts like a wash for the trapped dirt. There is also a broom provided in the form of longer hairs called 'cilia' that sweep the contaminated mucous into the throat so that it is swallowed by us and destroyed by acid in the stomach. If there is too much pollution or an allergy, there is over production of mucous and all of it cannot be swept away fast enough for swallowing, leading to blockage inside the nose and dribbling.

FIGHTING INFECTIONS

Nose also contains 'lysozymes' that fight bacteria, which enter it through the air. This is why although we inhale numerous viruses and bacteria; they do not infect us unless they are too many to be handled by the nose, or our immunity is low.

SENSE OF SMELL

Because of our eyes and ears, our sense of smell has not been utilised to its full potential. Actually, most people, objects, and areas can be recognised by smell. Visually and hearing impaired people demonstrate this capacity. Incidentally, there are some old time doctors who can 'smell out' patients of typhoid, liver failure, tuberculosis, and kidney failure!

How do we perceive smell? On the roof of the nose, there is a small patch of tissue with a few projecting hairs and millions of 'receptors' that receive the different smells. - All smells or odours probably consist of molecules that enter the nose and are 'received' by these receptors when they are swept onto them by the hairs. These receptors convey the information through the 'olfactory' nerve to the brain, which then recognises that we have smelt a 'rose' or a bad odour. Incidently we wrinkle our nose and turn away from a bad odour, to probably reduce the number of foul smelling molecules that can enter our nose. We also tend to develop immunity to bad odours if exposed long enough like workers who work in the atmosphere of smelly chemicals.

SNEEZING

Sneezing occurs when foreign particles irritate the nose, releasing chemical called histamine which irritates the nerves triggering a response that we call a sneeze.

The function of sneezing is to expel mucus containing foreign particles or irritants and cleanse the nasal cavity. During a sneeze, the soft palate and uvula depress while the back of the tongue elevates to partially close the passage to the mouth so that air ejected from the lungs may be expelled through the nose. Because the closing of the mouth is partial, a considerable amount of this air is usually also expelled from the mouth.

Most people would like to stop their sneezes, but it is mostly harmless to the individual. However infectious droplets of up to 40,000 in number and reaching several meters are shot out when a person sneezes, and this can lead to spread of infection when an infected person sneezes hard. I also remember a patient of mine who said everything was fine with her except she wanted to sneeze, but could not! Along with my colleagues I tried many conventional and some unconventional things but alas I could not help her! Now continuing with the serious part -

Can a sneeze be prevented?

Well you can try the following -

Hold your breath and slowly count to ten

- Crinkle your nose

- Pinch the bridge of the nose and hold for several seconds

Management

Stay away from irritants, and treat the cause. Anti histaminics can be taken in severe cases.

NOSE BLEEDS

Sometimes our body gets so heated up and the blood vessels expand so much, that they burst and we develop a nosebleed. This occurs more often in summer; but it can also happen in winter due to drying up and formation of cracks inside the nose. Nose bleed can be controlled by applying an ice pack, pinching the nostrils, packing it with a gauze soaked in Vaseline (petroleum jelly), and if really required, contracting the blood vessels with nasal drops or even oral drugs. Severe nosebleed can also be due to high blood pressure, some drugs like aspirin, or a bleeding disorder. In these conditions, the cause has to be treated.

NASAL POLYPS

These are small protuberances on the inner lining of the nose. If they are too large, they have to be removed by surgery to relieve the blocking.

DEVIATED SEPTUM

this is a condition in which there is a shift of the partition wall between the two nostrils to one side, thus reducing the size of one nostril. If it leads to excessive blockage, it has to be surgically corrected.

SINUSITIS, AND RHINITIS

Here there is inflammation in the nose and the sinuses. It can be due to an infection or an allergy. Breathing exercises, some nasal drops and sprays can help, along with a short course of antibiotics if needed.

A few things you should know -

NASAL DROPS

They cause temporary contraction of blood vessels, thus reducing secretions; but they can have a rebound effect-that is there can be an outpouring of secretions when the effect of the drops wears off. If used for too long they can also lead to permanent narrowing of blood vessels that can interfere with nasal functioning. There are also steroid containing nasal sprays that have a local anti-inflammatory effect.

BLOWING HARD ON THE NOSE

Never blow too hard on your nose; it can cause the eardrums to burst, leading to infection entering the sinuses and ears.

✦✦✦✦

8

Problems of Bones, Muscles and Joints

It happens to all of us - that sudden 'catch' in the back, a sprain, a fracture or even arthritis. The older concept of 'laid back' approach to these problems is gradually being replaced by early mobilisation, and newer techniques are being developed every year to achieve this.

To prevent any chronic problem from developing, we should literally bend backwards to keep our joints and spine supple. In the acute stages of pain, ice application should always be the first aid of choice, followed by immobilisation of the part. Heat treatment should only be started after forty-eight hours and not before. Now let us discuss a few common joint and bone problems-

OSTEOPOROSIS:

porous bone or thinning of bone is a very common problem of ageing. In healthy people bone is being constantly remodeled with addition and removal of matter to maintain a balance. Around menopause, bone loss exceeds bone formation, which leads to a negative balance with thinning of bone and increased incidence of fractures. However after sixty, osteoporosis is equally seen in both sexes.

What are the factors that influence osteoporosis?

These can be: -

1) Sex hormone deficiency- there are some oestrogen receptors in the bones, which help in uptake of calcium in the presence of female hormones. Supplementing oestrogens from outside or giving natural oestrogens in the form of Soya, helps in these cases.

2) Calcium status- our body needs about 800 milligrams of calcium daily and after menopause this doubles. Good dietary sources of calcium are greens and dairy products.

3) Physical activity- exercise, especially yoga and weight bearing exercises influence bone growth in a positive way.

4) Drugs – like steroids or thyroid hormones can cause thinning of bones.

5) Diseases- like hyperthyroidism, hyperparathyroidism, spread of cancer to bones, certain diseases of bones, and kidney diseases can all cause osteoporosis.

What are the factors, which indicate risk of fractures?

These can be-

1) Increase of certain enzymes in blood called alkaline phosphatase

2) X-ray showing thinning of bone

3) Bone scan (after injecting radioactive material) showing hair-line cracks

4) Bone densimetry- SXA (single energy x-ray) or DEXA (double energy x-ray)-shows bone thinning.

5) Bone biopsy- directly reveals bone thinning.

6) C.T. scan---it can also reveal thinning of bones.

Guidelines for management of Osteoporosis

1) Supplementation with calcium and vitamin –D.

2) Hormone replacement

3) Drugs like - Biphosphonates

   Calcitonin

   Sodium fluoride

   Anabolic steroids

   Parathormone

   Biologicals

4) Exercise -   Yoga and load bearing exercises (with weights)

Guidelines for prevention of Fractures

1) Using sticks

2) Making bathrooms and staircases safe

3) Wearing proper glasses

4) Ensuring good lighting

ARTHRITIS

Arthritis can be osteoarthritis (arthritis of old age) or due to various other causes like infections, reaction to infections, rheumatoid, rheumatic, metabolic – (gout) etc. When you suffer from Arthritis – try to find out any curable cause like infective (tuberculosis, gonorhoea, syphilis) or metabolic (gout, rheumatoid) reaction to infection (like rheumatic) etc. before concluding that it is degenerative arthritis of old age called osteoarthritis.

A word of caution: -

Rheumatoid arthritis is a group of arthritis, which should be treated intensively – otherwise joint damage can occur.

RHEUMATOID ARTHRITIS

Rheumatoid arthritis is one of a group of diseases called 'auto-immune diseases' in which the body's immune system turns against itself. Immune system is the system that protects us from internal and external agents that can cause disease. Normally the immune system recognizes the body's tissues as 'self' and fights against all 'non-self' or foreign tissues by the formation of *antibodies*. But in *auto immune diseases*, the immune system fails to make this distinction and fights against 'self' tissues also, resulting in their destruction Let us try to understand this process. Foreign tissues like viruses, bacteria, other organisms and agents are regularly attacking the body. These harmful agents are called *antigens*. In order to protect itself from repeated attacks from these agents, the body develops protective chemicals called *antibodies*. These antibodies now act as guards and if there is a re-invasion by the harmful aggressors, they fight and destroy them. In Rheumatoid arthritis, how the process is triggered is not known, but certain bacteria (streptococci) or viruses may be responsible. This *autoimmune* process results in inflammation in various parts of the body including joints and muscles.

In *Rheumatoid arthritis*, joints are involved symmetrically unlike in other forms of arthritis. Later, other parts of the body can be affected, like eyes, heart, lungs, skin (nodule formation), nerves, blood vessels, spleen and lymph nodes. RA afflicts 1% of the population. The disease is common all over the world but is seen less in black Africans. Some have a mild self-limiting disease that is totally cured, in most it is slowly progressive, but in a few, the disease can have a hectic course with rapid progression.

It is more prevalent in women, with a preponderance of 3:1 over men. Disease onset is most common in middle age though children and the old can also develop new disease. The majority of patients develop joint damage within 2 years of disease onset, and maximum progression of erosion and joint space narrowing occurs within the first few years. *Therefore the modern concept is to vigorously treat the disease as soon as it is diagnosed especially in severe cases* with 'disease modifying anti- rheumatic drugs or DMARDS', steroids, and newer drugs called 'biologicals' to save the joint from damage.

GOUT:

It is a condition where excessive uric acid in the blood gets deposited in the joints, leading to severe pain, redness and swelling. It is seen in people consuming a protein rich diet and also alcohol. It is thus also called "a disease of kings and a king of diseases" Reduction in intake of alcohol, proteins and intake of certain drugs helps in reducing uric acid in the blood, and some anti inflammatory drugs help in taking care of the pain and swelling.

OSTEOARTHRITIS

Before discussing osteoarthritis, we should understand what a joint consists of - As the name suggests, **a joint** is the joining of two or more bones to make the limb mobile or flexible. Let us take the example of the knee in which the femur or thighbone joins with the tibia and fibula from the leg, to form a joint.

The knee joint has a **joint space**, covered by a **capsule,** two **opposing surfaces of the bone** which are covered with **cartilage,** the capsule itself being lined by **synovial membrane** from inside, which secretes lubricating fluid, thus preventing wear and tear. The joint is supported from the outside by **muscles,** which are attached to the bone by means of a **tendon.** Contraction and relaxation of muscles is responsible for movement at the joint. **Ligaments** are structures that join two bones to each other. Now that our basics are clear, we can understand arthritis better.

Osteoarthritis is a disease of ageing, which affects all of us to a greater or lesser extent. It normally begins after 45 years of age and is commoner in ladies. Some people are genetically predisposed to a severe form of the disease, and in some it can start at an earlier age due to certain birth defects. Lack of female hormones, muscle weakness, trauma and obesity can hasten the process of osteoarthritis, and imbalance in certain minerals like calcium and phosphorous, thyroid problems, and uric acid deposition in the joint also accelerates osteoarthritis. Now what are the changes that occur inside the joint in osteoarthritis?

Front view of Normal Knee

Joint changes:

Joint changes there maybe thinning of the cartilage, thickening of joint surface, microscopic fractures, thinning of bone, new bone formation, loose bodies inside the joint, weakening of the muscles, swelling and fluid accumulation. These changes lead to pain, swelling and restricted mobility of the joint. Now how do we manage osteoarthritis?

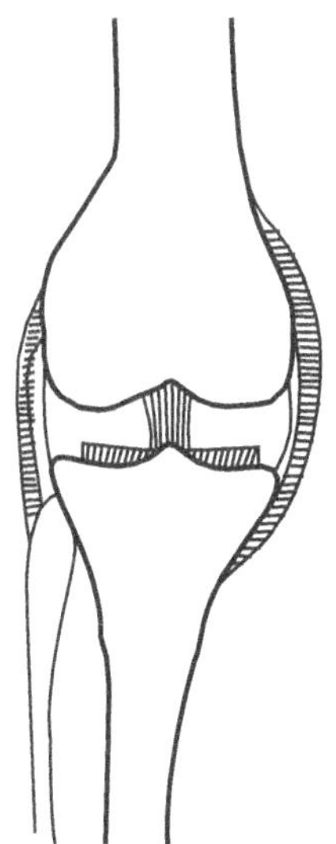

Guidelines for Management

+ Control obesity

+ Treat pain with drugs, hot wax and other measures

+ Walking stick and shock absorbing insoles in shoes to avoid strain on the joint

+ Injections inside joint to reduce swelling

+ Surgery

Surgery itself can be of various types:

1) Repairing the joint by removing loose bodies, trimming frayed cartilage, etc; using an arthroscope (a self-illuminating instrument with cutting ends where the joint can be visualized and minor procedures performed without a big incision)

2) Repairing the joint with open surgery

3) Partial joint replacement

4) Full joint replacement

In full joint replacement, the joint surfaces are replaced with an artificial one made of metal and polypropylene. Pain is immediately reduced, but sitting on the floor cross-legged is not possible, and life of the new joint is about ten years. Newer joints are said to enable sitting cross-legged on the floor.

SPINE

"We are as young as our spine", so if you keep your spine flexible and supple, you will remain young even at eighty! Keep bending that spine forwards, backwards and sideways, preferably under supervision of a good yoga teacher (or continue to sweep, swab, dust, wash clothes and do housework at full stretch!) Any severe problem of the spine can only be corrected by exercise. Rest is needed only in the acute stage when pain is severe, so *start moving* as soon as possible and enter a good exercise program, or the axiom will hold true of "once a backache, always a backache". Now let us discuss a very common problem called spondylitis.

SPONDYLITIS

Spondylitis is a process of aging which all of us undergo to a greater or lesser extent. It tends to affect the cervical (neck) and lumbar (lower back) more than the rest of the spine since these parts are more mobile and hence subjected to more stress. Nature has given good protection to our spinal cord, in the form of,

1) A bony cage formed by vertebra

2) A strong muscular support

3) A good cushion in the form of inter-vertebral discs

Brain and Spinal Cord   Spine

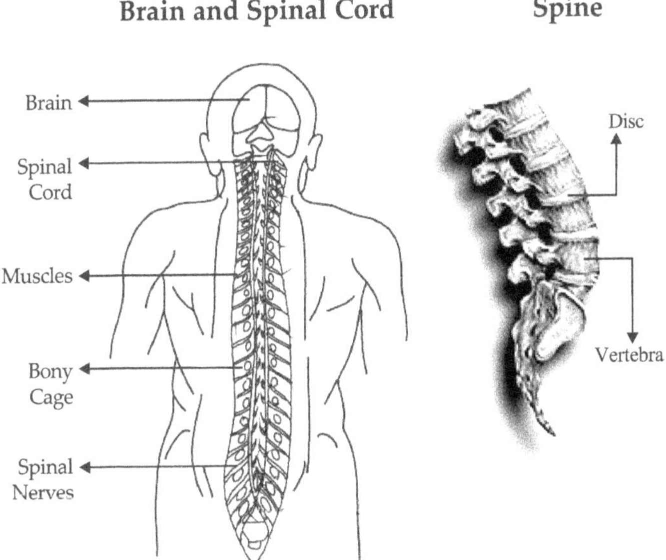

This protection if supplemented by a good diet and moderate exercise, can keep our spines supple even life-long; but if we neglect it, spondylitic changes can be hastened. Now let us see what happens to our spines in spondylitis: -

Changes in spondylitis are due to repeated stress that our spine is subjected to.

1) The disc between the vertebrae becomes thin and weak, and intervertebral space reduces. Sometimes, the disc may even prolapse outwards, or inwards, thus pressing on the spinal nerves or even the cord.

2) Bony outgrowths may occur leading to pressure on nerves.

All these changes lead to various complaints like pain, tingling, numbness, and if the cord is affected, even paralysis. Since spine is an organ of balance, anything which affects it can cause imbalance and giddiness, and sometimes when a nerve root is compressed, the patient may be gripped in a vice like grip of pain called *root pain*. *Sciatica* another common condition we hear about is due to pressure on the sciatic nerve in the lower back. Now how can we slow down this process of spondylitis?

Prevention of progress

This can be achieved by various means-

1) Posture correction Sitting with a pillow behind the small of the back, helps to prevent a "slump" in the posture and thus strain on the lower spine. This can also be achieved by using a good chair.

2) Intermittent neck and foot exercises during working hours will prevent stiffness from developing.

3) A good exercise program must be adhered to.

4) A balanced diet with plenty of greens, dairy products and fruits ensures adequate supply of calcium, and other minerals which are essential for a healthy spine, especially if it is accompanied by exposure to sunlight, which helps in converting vitamin D to its active form.

Supposing spondylitis has developed, how do we manage it?

Management of Spondylitis

This is done by various techniques-

1) Rest

2) Immobilisation with collar, belts etc. These should be for a short term only and not continued life-long.

3) Drugs for pain, swelling and giddiness- again only for a short time.

4) Some other methods of relieving pain like deep ray treatment, by using electric currents, etc.

5) Physiotherapy and traction.

6) Surgery

Surgery

There are various surgical techniques, which help in spondylitis. We can remove bony outgrowths, trim prolapsed parts of disc, thus relieving compression of the cord and nerves, or we can even fuse the joints together after relieving the compression to avoid further friction and pain.

Some techniques in management of bones and joints you may like to know about

1. **Ilizarov techniqe:** is for fractures where the person need not be immobilised. It is useful for fractures of legs and was developed by a Russian doctor. It involves a series of horizontal and vertical supports, which are screwed up from outside, to immobilise the limb. It is light, effective and best of all, the patient is mobile and since no plaster is used, the limb feels lighter.

3 **Joint Injections** with hyaluronic acid may lessen pain and swelling of the affected joint.

4 **Cartilage transplant**: Now a piece of your own cartilage can be extracted, grown outside the body and these new extra cells can be reinserted by another minor operation. Soon a new layer of cartilage may form if all goes well.

Alternatively a large piece of cartilage may be removed from an unimportant joint and transplanted.

Finally, a few easy exercises have been included for those of you who do not know them already. Do them regularly and you can be like old father William, turning cartwheels at eighty!

EXERCISES:

All exercises should be done slowly and the positions maintained for some time for maximum efficacy and also to avoid any damage to the body.

CALF & ANKLES

Push against
the wall

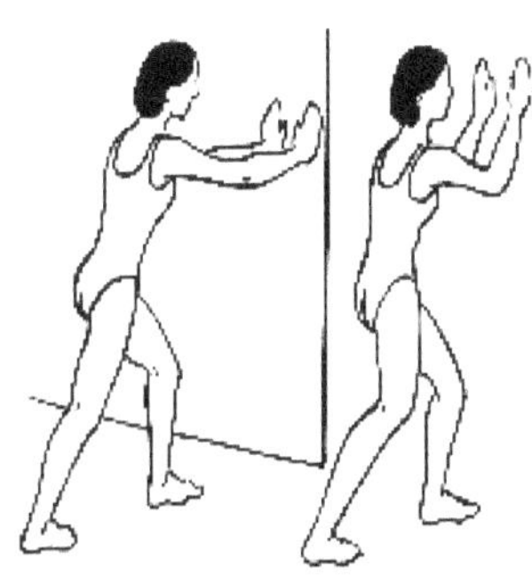

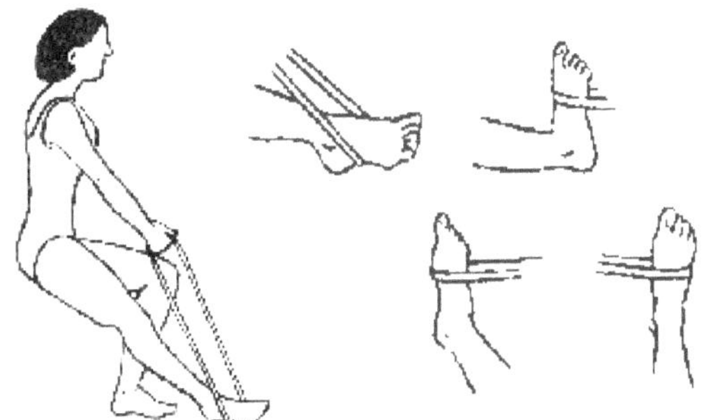

Pull with rope - up, down, side to side

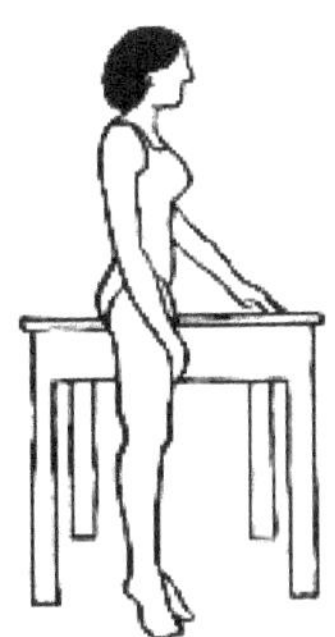

Stand on toes at
full stretch with
hand on table
for support

NECK and SPONDYLITIS

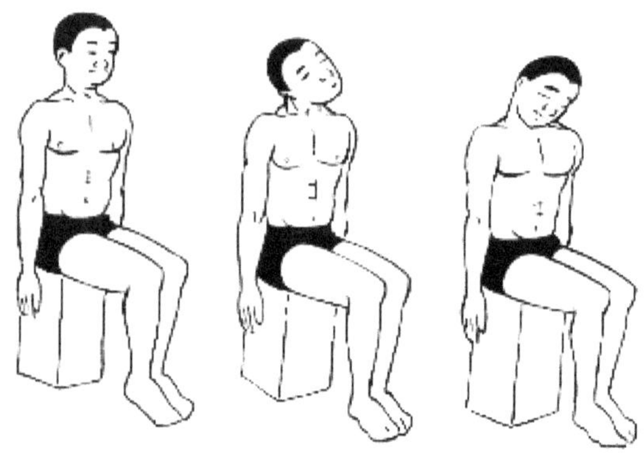

Bend head to right side,
touch shoulder & repeat on left side.

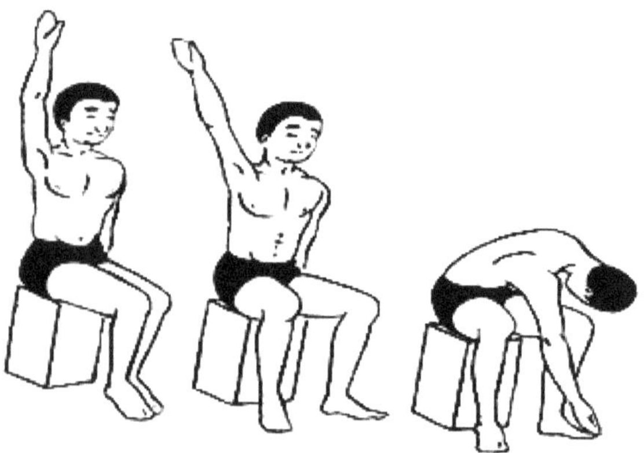

Raise right hand & turn it backwards, following the hand with
head & eyes. Now bend hand down & touch the left foot with
it while touching fore head to left knee. Do the same with left
hand, right foot and right knee

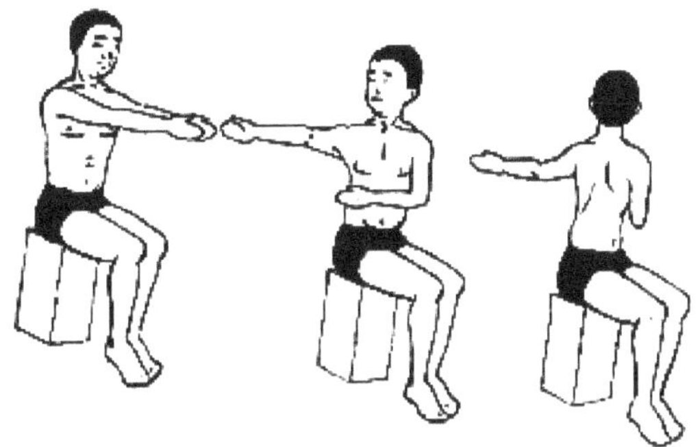

Move both hands forwards then slowly move right hand to right, now slowly turn to left spreading out left hand and folding right, while keeping lower part of body fixed. Repeat with left hand.

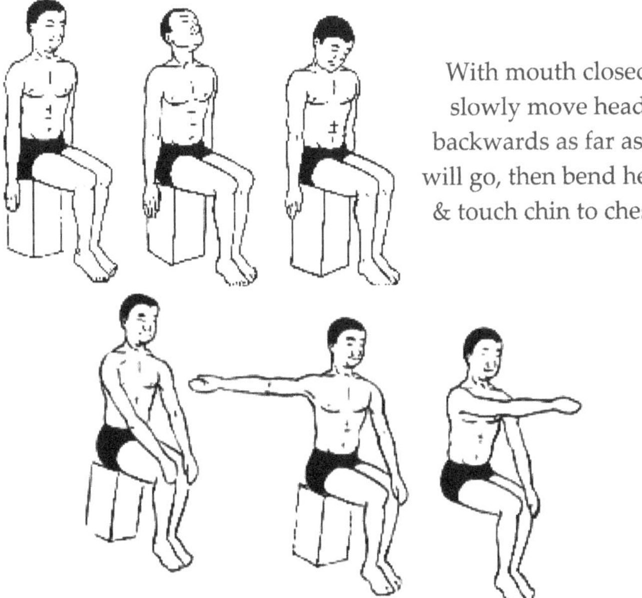

With mouth closed slowly move head backwards as far as it will go, then bend head & touch chin to chest.

Keep hands spread out, twist to right keeping lower part of body still. Now repeat on left side.

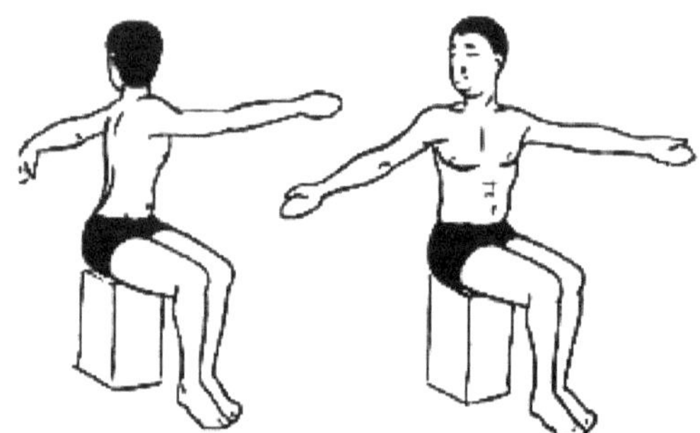

Keep both hands on knees. Move right hand to the right then forward and down. Repeat with left hand.

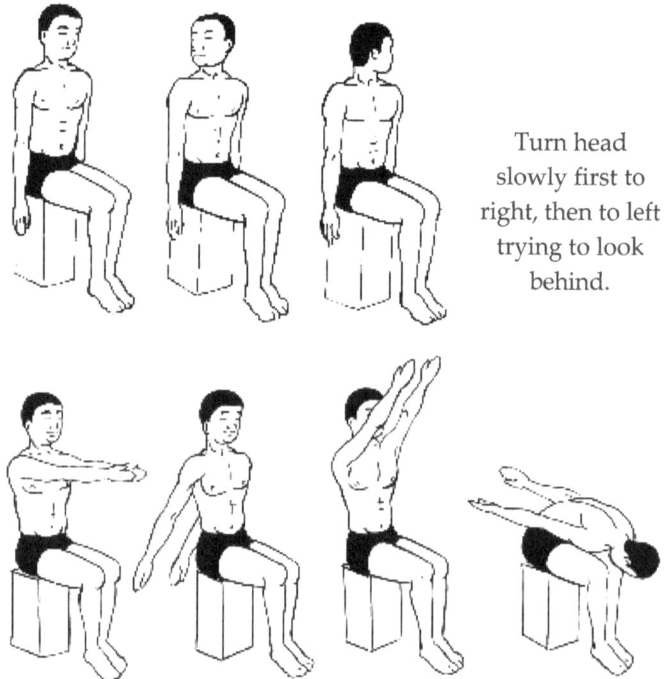

Turn head slowly first to right, then to left trying to look behind.

Move both hands backwards, then slowly forwards. Now bend head & touch it to knees & at the same time move hands back slowly.

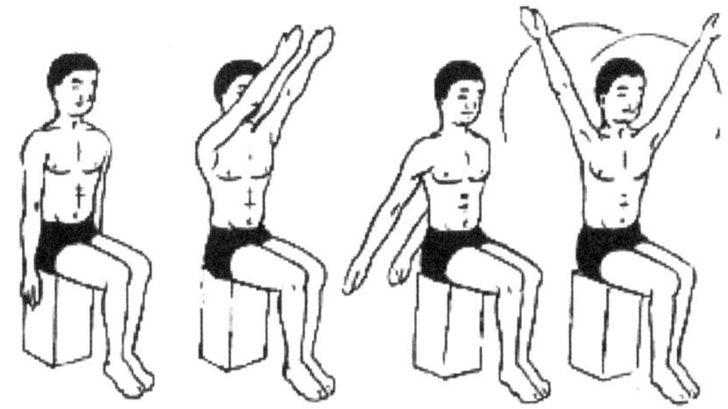

Move hands forwards, backwards, & rotate slowly.

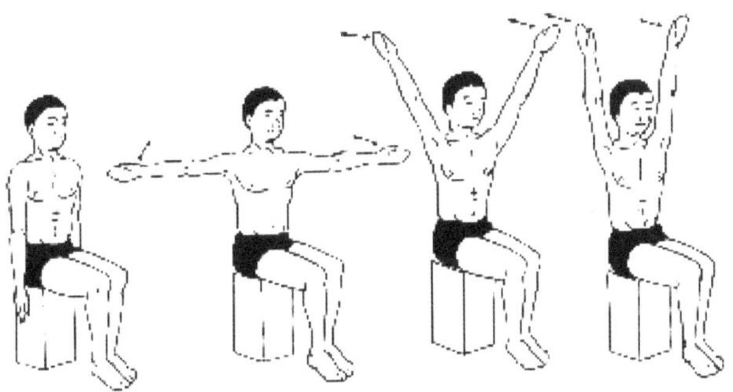

Spread both hands and then move them slowly upwards to touch ears and back.

SHOULDER

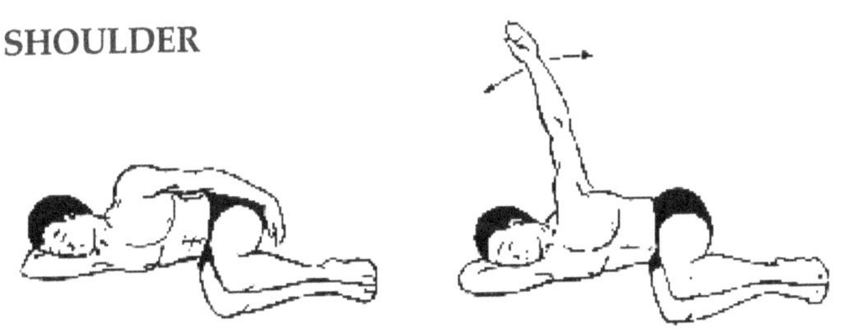

Lie down as shown on one side, raise upper hand sideways, bend & touch ear keeping hand straight at elbow then take it back. Do the same with the other hand.

Problems of Bones, Muscles and Joints

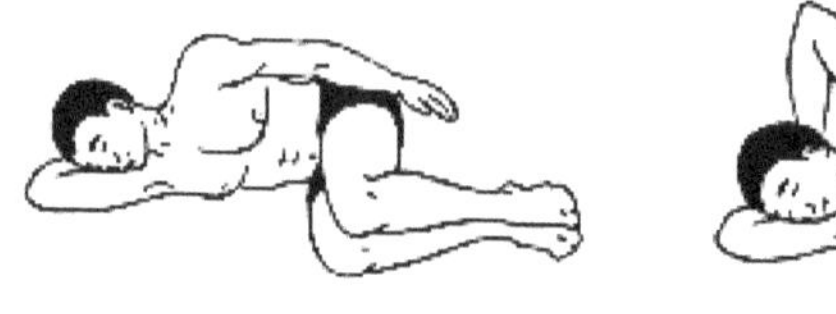
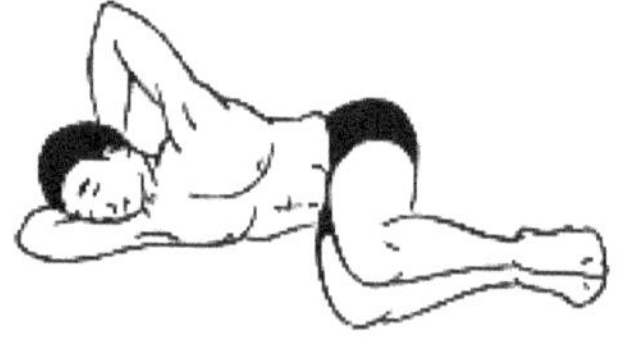

Lie on healthy side, raise arm straight up & bring the hand behind the head as shown then again straighten hand & bring to starting position.

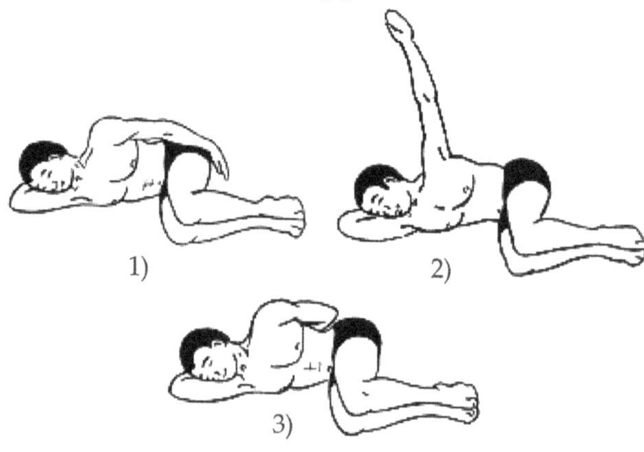

Move the forearm across the shoulder and behind the back as shown in picture 1,2, & 3.

STANDING

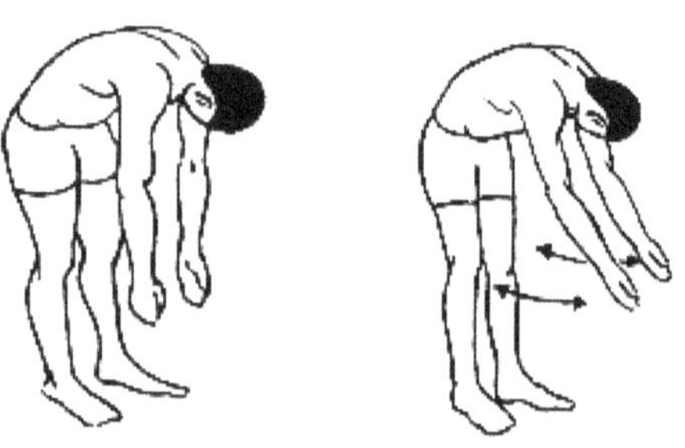

Bend down & swing arms forwards & backwards

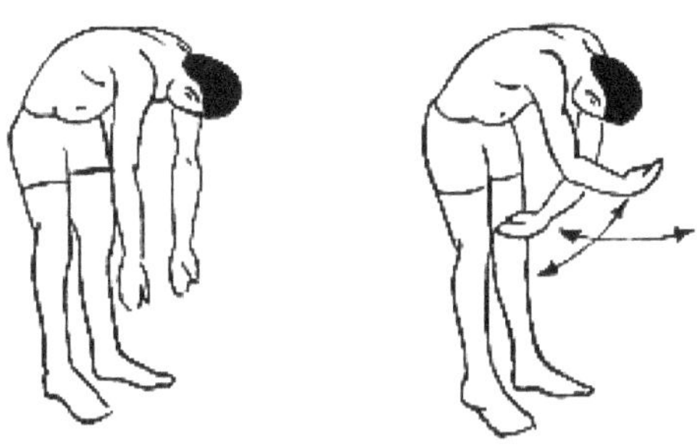

Swing arms sideways as shown.

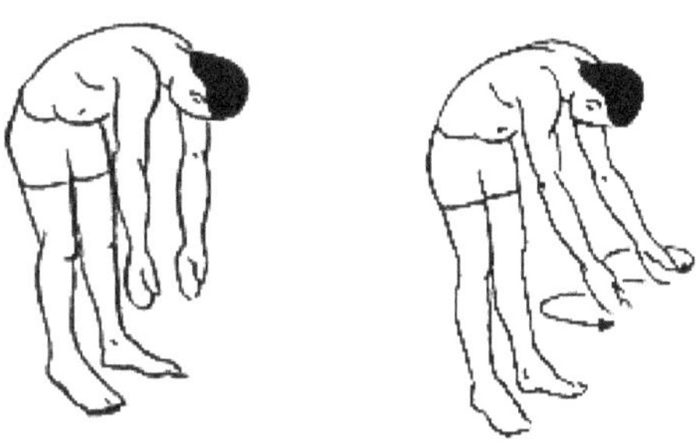

Describe small circles with the arms.

KNEES

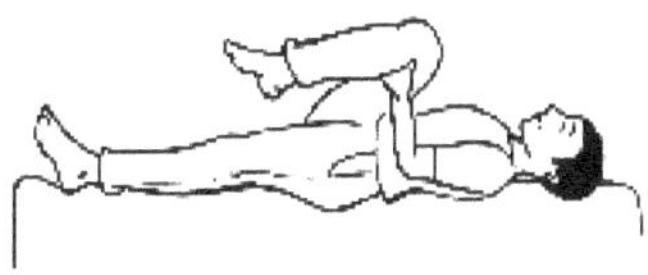

LYING DOWN

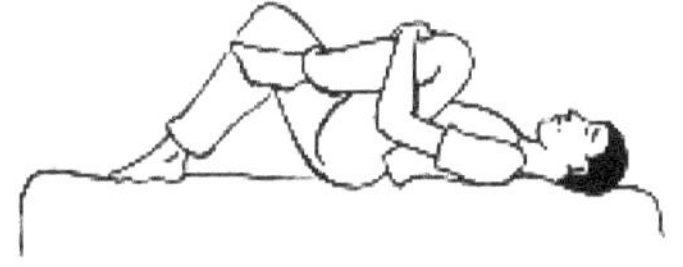

Lie down on ground, bend one knee, touch chest & straighten,
keeping other leg against wall. Repeat with the other leg.

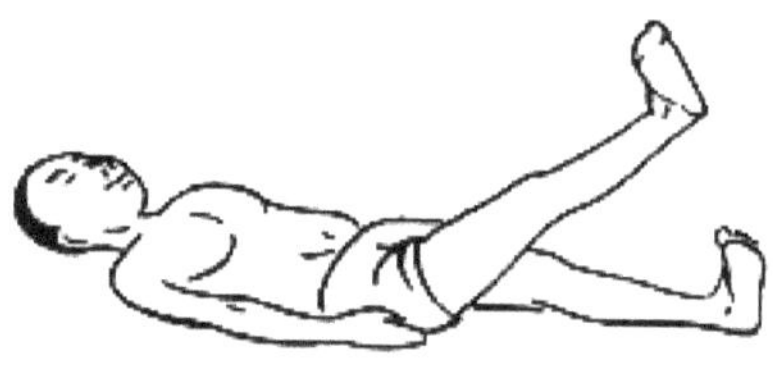

Lift one leg straight up to 45 degrees & down very slowly.

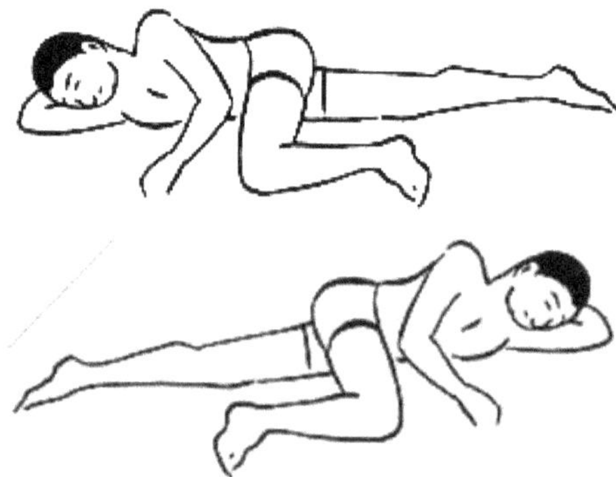

Lying down on right side bend left leg at knee & straighten.
Now repeat with right leg lying on left side.

SITTING

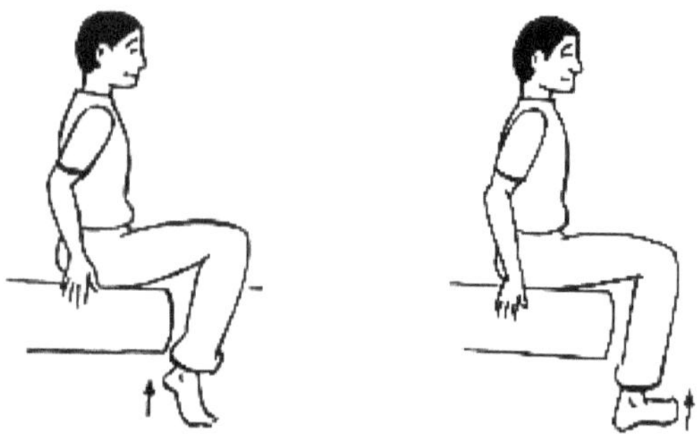

Sitting on chair press down firmly on its arms alternately
raising ankles & toes, as slowly as possible.

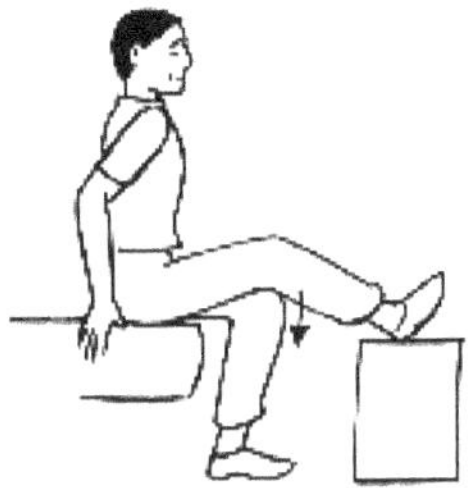

Rest one leg straight on block and press down.
Repeat with the other leg.

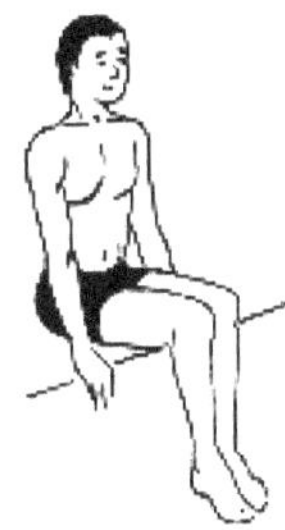 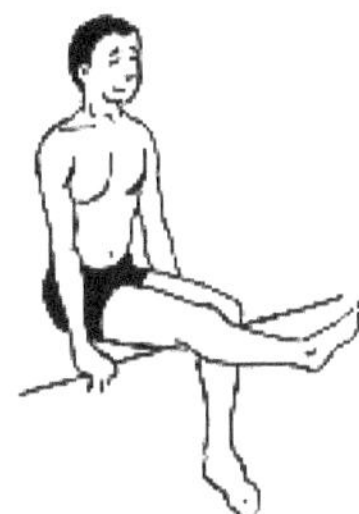

Sitting on a chair or bench lift one leg at a time
straight up & down slowly.

STANDING

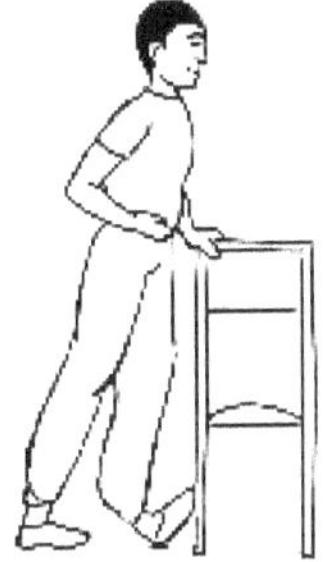 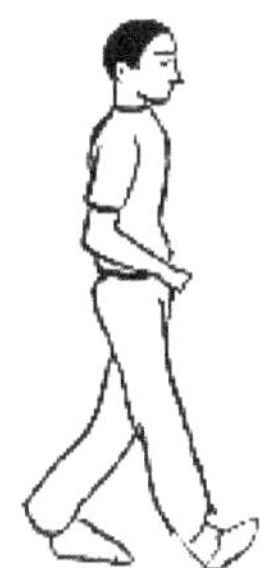

Stand near stool or chair keep
one foot against leg of stool
pointing up for some time
then repeat with the other foot

Walk in a straight line on
your right ankle (with toes
raised) Repeat exercise
walking on left ankle.

WRISTS

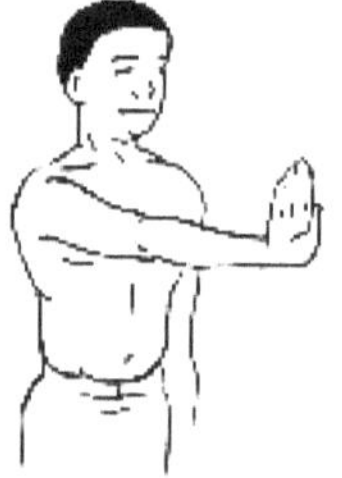

Stand with your hand outstretched palm touching wall and press against it. Repeat with other hand.

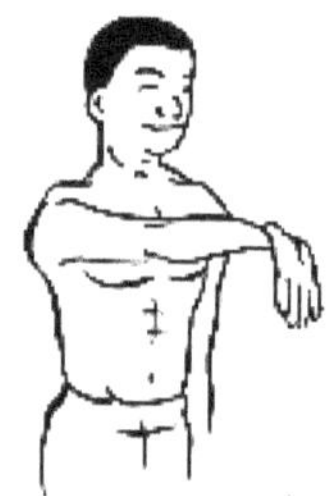

Lift right arm to shoulder height palm facing up, spread fingers and bend wrist downwards.

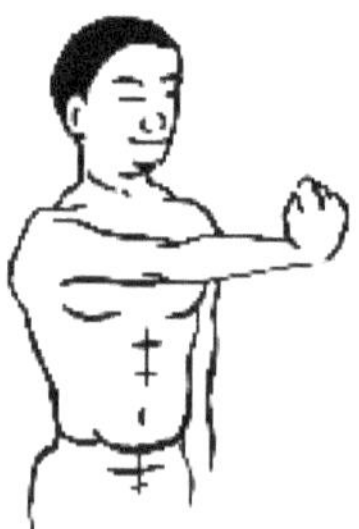

Keeping arm extended make a fist and bend wrist upwards.

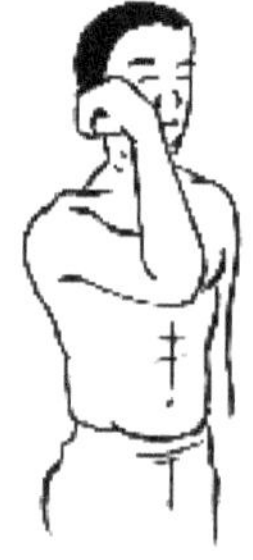

With bent elbow, bring fist towards shoulder.

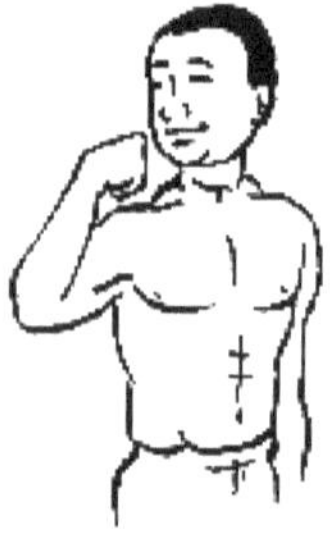

Rotate elbow to side and look at fist.

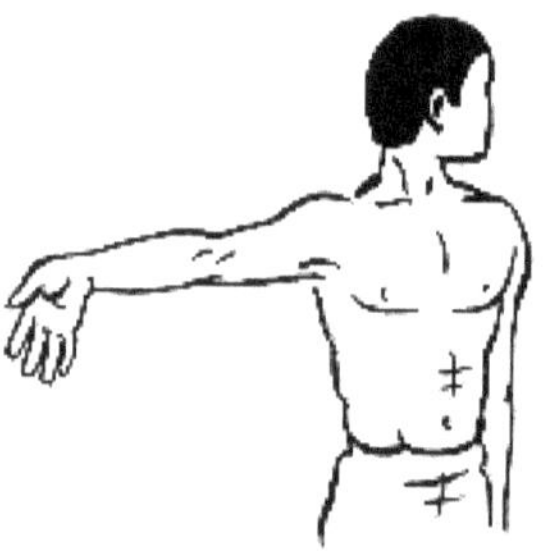

With outstretched hand spread fingers and bend wrist downwards, while slowly turning towards opposite side.

BACK

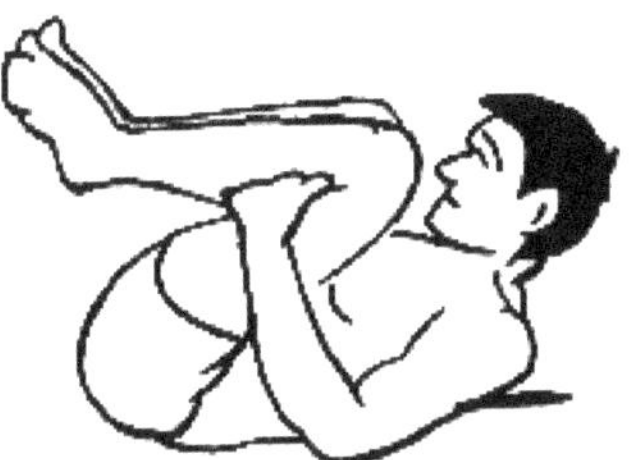

Pull both legs up and fold over stomach, grip behind knees,
now lift shoulders and try to roll from side to side.

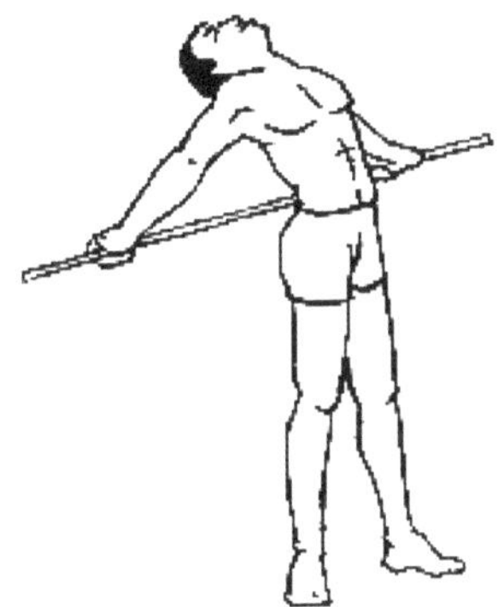

Press a smooth bamboo against lower part of back as shown
and slowly bend upper part of body backwards as shown,
maintain for some time and come back.

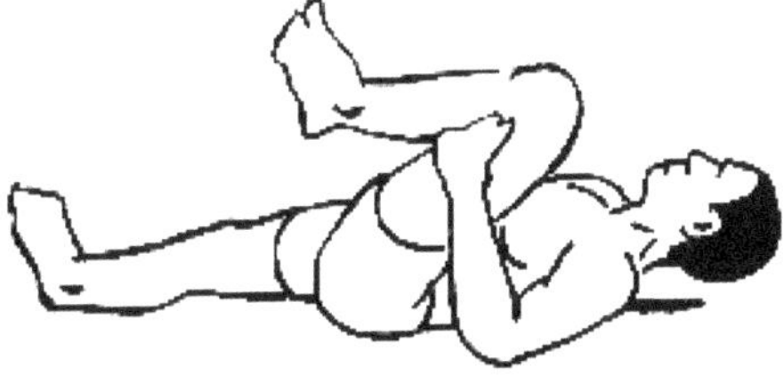

Lie on back with one knee bent and the other flat on floor.
Now flex both feet, grip bent leg behind knee, and pull toward
chest, to feel stretch in buttocks and lower back. Repeat with
other leg.

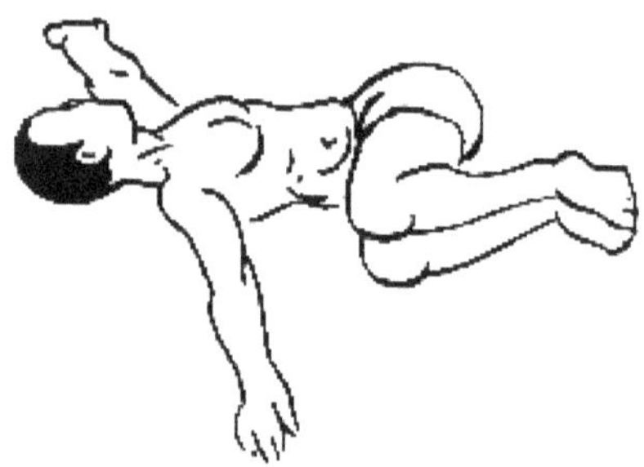

Lie on back with knees bent feet touching floor, and head
turned to left. Now bring knees to chest, and slowly let them fall
to the right till they rest on the floor, and hold for 10 seconds.
Come back to original position and repeat on other side.

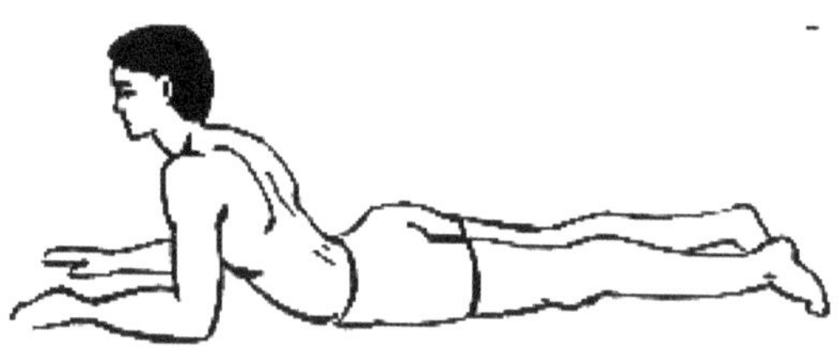

Lie on stomach with upper body propped up on forearms,
press pelvis down and hold for two minutes. Now push upper
body higher by straightening arms and return to original
position.

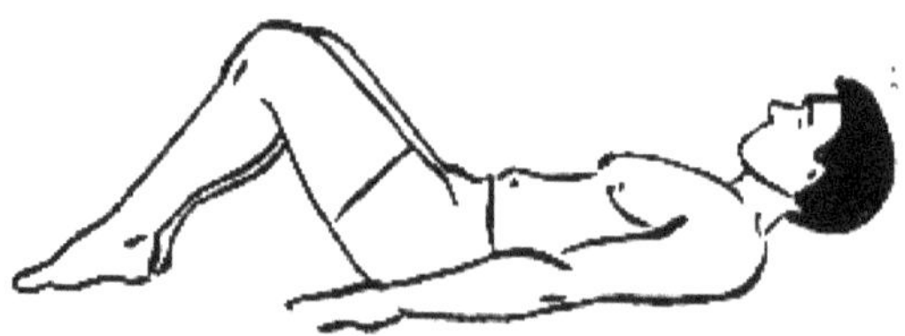

Lie on back with knees bent, palms facing down, lift your head
and shoulders slowly count three and come back to original
position.

Management of bony & muscular pains

R- Rest

I- Ice

C- Compression

E- Elevation

CHECKLIST OF COMMON CAUSES OF BACKACHE

1. Postural, due to wrong methods of sitting or standing
2. Deformities in spine
3. Sprain or derangement due to lifting heavy weights or fall
4. Fracture of spine or hip
5. Slipped disc
6. Compression of nerve
7. Tuberculosis of spine or other infections
8. Cancer of spine
9. In ladies, due to periods or inflammation in pelvis
10. Prostatic problems
11. Urinary problems
12. Ulcer in duodenum (upper intestines)
13. Kidney and gall stones
14. Infection or inflammation in any organ in abdomen
15. Problems of uterus, tubes and ovaries
16. Fissure and piles
17. Some diseases of muscles
18. After injections in spine for anaesthesia
19. Arthritis of spine
20. Psychiatric causes

+ + + +

9

Skin

Skin is the largest organ of the human body, and performs many important functions like protecting us from dust, bacteria, air, and water, eliminating waste matter, regulating and maintaining body temperature, and giving us the sense of touch. It is composed of cells which keep dying and are being renewed all the time, so, the skin you have today is not the same one you had last year! Like our eyes, skin also reflects the state of our internal health so a well-toned and glowing skin generally denotes an excellent constitution. Though nature has designed it to maintain itself, a well-balanced diet, daily cleaning and skin care, fresh air, regular exercise, nutritious food, sufficient sleep and mental stability are the essential factors for the maintenance of a supple and healthy skin.

The thickness and sensitivity of skin also varies from person to person and usually, female skin has more fat, which gives a soft and rounded look to the body.

Skin consists of two major layers. The superficial layer is called *epidermis* and the inner layer is called *dermis*. The epidermis is made up of several rows of living cells covered with a horny layer of dead cells. The epidermis protects the inner layer. In the basal layer of the epidermis are cells which produce a pigment, called *melanin*. Melanin guards the skin against sunlight and determines the colour of the skin. In fact darker the skin, the more resistant it is to harmful effects of sun, especially to skin cancer.

 Dermis is the living layer and it contains supporting tissues, which gives the skin its tone and resilience. It also contains the sweat and oil glands, blood vessels and lymphatics. The sebaceous glands, which produce oil known as sebum, keep the skin supple, and lubricate it, while its acid content resists bacterial attacks and keeps the skin in a healthy condition.

STRUCTURE OF THE SKIN

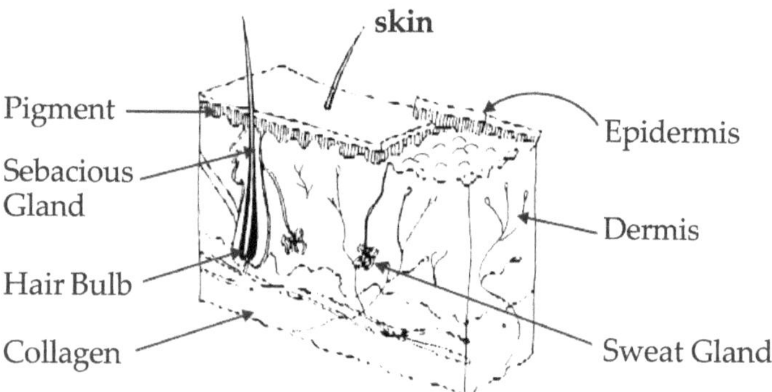

Sweat glands help to eliminate wastes and regulate body temperature, capillary blood vessels supply oxygen and nutrients to the skin, and lymphatic vessels drain away waste products. The hair roots lie beneath the skin.

SKIN CARE

It is essential to know your skin type for choosing the right skin care treatment. An easy way to discover what type of skin you have is to wipe your face with a dry tissue early in the morning soon after you leave your bed. If there is oil on it, you have 'greasy' skin. If you have grease only on your forehead and nose, you have a 'combination' skin. If there is no grease on the tissue at all, then you have either a dry skin or a normal one.

SKIN – TYPES

Normal Skin

A healthy normal skin is unblemished, velvety, smooth and glowing. It has no enlarged pores. To maintain it in this ideal state, it needs care like daily cleaning, toning, nourishing, and massaging.

Oily Skin

The sebaceous glands are over-active, produce more oil than is needed, thus making the face greasy and enlarging the pores, with black heads and acne. Grease tends to pile up dirt and grime, which clog the pores and produce black heads. Therefore, oily skin needs special cleaning to keep the pores unclogged.

Dry Skin

This skin lacks both sebum and moisture. It has dry patches and cracks. Cold weather, exposure to sun, air, air-conditioners, as well as frequent washing with soap and water are the factors, which accentuate dry skin and cause wrinkles and lines.

Dry skin needs care to prevent premature ageing.

Sensitive Skin

Intense cold and heat has a bad effect on this type of skin. Sensitive skin also reacts to internal problems in the body.

Skin constantly undergoes changes depending on weather conditions, environmental pollution, tension, insomnia, use of tranquillisers, sun and wind, all of which accelerate the ageing process. We can retard this process by taking good care of our skin.

DAILY REGIME FOR THE SKIN

These guidelines also help in protecting, preventing and correcting any skin problems. Daily regime is a matter of habit like brushing the teeth, bathing, adequate sleep, proper diet and exercise.

1) Massage -

massage your body with oil regularly. In

winter, warm the oil before use.

Body massage has many advantages. It gives relief from pain and fatigue, makes the skin and muscles healthy and strong, increases immunity, and is good for the eyes.

If whole body massage is not possible daily, then at least massage the head and bottom of the feet, or massage the whole body once a week. Exercise at least for 10 to 15 minutes after the massage.

The next step is to massage the body again with the help of scrubs (use any flour) to remove oil from the body, dead cells from the skin, and to melt fat accumulated under the skin. The regimen of massage also energises the mind.

Cleansing

Cleansing is required for removing oil, dust, perspiration, dirt, bacteria etc. because all these collect on your skin and must be removed completely.

CLEANSING HERBS	TYPE OF SKIN
Sandalwood	Oily
Neem	Oily
Rose	Medium
Papaya	Medium
Strawberry	Dry skin
Fenugreek	Medium
Aloe vera	Dry skin
Turmeric	Oily skin

Useful Tips

+ Aloe, papaya, strawberry, and carrot are re-hydrating cleansers

+ **For a dry skin** – Instead of soap, one can use oatmeal or almond meal. Cleansing should be done with a cream followed by a very mild tonic like rose water

+ Turmeric has healing properties and lightens the skin colour

TONING

Toning stimulates blood supply to the skin. Weekly toning treatments help to revitalize the skin and get rid of wrinkles and lines.

Toning Herbs	Type of skin
Rose	Any type
Marigold	Any type
Aloe Vera	Dry
Orange	Oily
Lime	Oily
Sesame oil	Dry
Coconut oil	Any type
Mustard oil	Oily

MOISTURISING AND NOURISHING THE SKIN

Skin needs moisture, which helps to freshen and soften the outer skin.

Moisturisers help to achieve a perfect balance of oil and moisture so that the skin is kept soft and smooth.

With the help of suitable cosmetic herbs, one can prevent the skin from drying up and ageing.

Moisturising Herbs	Type of skin
Almond	Dry, oily
Sunflower	Dry, oily
Aloe vera	Dry, oily
Rose	Dry, oily
Nutmeg	Oily
Saffron	Dry, oily
Coconut	Dry, oily
Lotus	Oily

Useful Tips

+ Rose water mixed with glycerin can be used as a moisturizer

+ Pulp of aloe can be used as moisturizer and as a sun screen

NOURISHING THE SKIN

The skin needs nourishment like the rest of the body, for sustaining its properties. Nourishing herbs are 'skin foods' which improve the skin's function- therefore they are found generally in our regular food like carrot, cabbage, wheat germs etc.

Skin requires amino acids (from proteins) for rebuilding, as there is constant shedding of dead cells, fatty acids for lubrication and vitamin A, vitamin C, iron, vitamin K, zinc, alpha hydroxy acids, and copper, to keep it fit. Sugarcane juice, buttermilk, citrus fruits, cucumber, apples, grapes and turmeric are excellent internal tonics for the skin, and along with sandal wood, also act as natural 'peelers' or 'exfoliators' when used externally.

NOURISHING HERBS FOR SKIN REJUVENATION
(TO BE TAKEN INTERNALLY)

+ Rose
+ sesame
+ almond
+ apricot
+ Liquorice

Useful Tips

+ Almond, and apricot contain vitamin A
+ Carrot and wheat germ are rich in vitamin E
+ Cabbage contains useful minerals for the skin

WOUND HEALING:

There are certain diseases and medicines which delay wound healing. So if you are taking any of the following medicines or suffering from these diseases, inform your doctor if you sustain an injury.

Medicines	Diseases
Steroids	Diabetes
Interferon	mental problems
Anticoagulants	AIDS
Immuno suppressants	Deficiency of vitamin C & zinc

HAIR PROBLEMS

Hair problems plague all of us, either too little, too much, or the wrong colour.

Greying

Greying has become easier to handle with all kinds of colouring aids available, but check out for allergies before using a new brand. There are some good herbs like, fenugreek, Indian gooseberry and henna which delay graying.

Excessive Hair

Excessive hair on the body bothers most ladies and usually there is no cause for it except in a few where hormonal imbalance of various types, can be responsible. These may be due to certain diseases like polycystic ovaries or drugs

Diseases	Drugs
Excessive male hormones	- steroids
Excessive prolactin (hormone)	- streptomycin
Hypothyroidism	- PUVA therapy
(less thyroidHormone)	(Ultraviolet ray therapy)
Malnutrition	
Malignancy (cancer)	Minoxidil etc.
Anorexia nervosa	

Management

Shaving, plucking, waxing, depilatory creams, electrolysis, and thermo blending, laser or photo depilation can remove excessive hair. The last three are permanent solutions. Oestrogens, anti-androgens, and many other drugs also help, but should be taken only under medical supervision

Baldness

Just as excessive hair normally bothers ladies, lack of it bothers men, especially on the head. Baldness may be due to:

Genetic Causes

- ✦ Hypothyrodiam
- ✦ Fungal diseases
- ✦ Alopecia areata
- ✦ Lupus Erythematosis
- ✦ Pyoderma (pus in skin)
- ✦ Lichen planus
- ✦ Psoriasis
- ✦ Mental problems especially a condition called Tricho - tilo - mania (literally pulling out one's own hair!)

Management of Baldness

1. Minoxidil cream (improvement in 30 – 40% cases)
2. Anti androgens – help in women with male pattern baldness
3. Hair weaving - existing hair is woven to cover bald area
4. Hair transplant - hair taken from dense area and transplanted to sparse area
5. Scalp reduction - reducing the bald patch to make it appear smaller
6. Sticking or clipping on tufts of artificial hair (shows remarkable results)
7. Wigs
8. Treating underlying disease

PIGMENT OR COLOUR PROBLEMS

Like hair, skin pigment may be too little or too much.

VITILIGO

Vitiligo is the commonest cause of 'white patches' or leucoderma, which may also be due to leprosy or fungal infections. Vitiligo is not a disease and the patient is only cosmetically affected. It can be managed with creams, oral drugs, and PUVA (light) therapy, tattooing or skin transplantation

Too much pigment – may be due to:

1. Hormonal imbalance – for example 'Melasma' or pregnancy mask on the face

2. Solar dermatitis

3. Freckles

4. Some cancers

Dark pigmentation can be treated with lightening creams or laser, and freckles and spots can be treated by *Dermabrasion* (discussed later)

SCARS

After burns or injuries, scars may be left, which may be pitted, or protuberant. These can be treated by *Cryo* surgery especially acne scars. Cryo is a process of freezing with carbon dioxide snow, or liquid nitrogen. The tissue dies metabolically and new skin is regenerated. For 6 weeks however, exposure to sunlight should be avoided. Cryo surgery is also used for other minor surgeries like removing *keloids* (overgrowth of tissue after burn or injury healing), *warts* (a viral infection leading to small growths), or moles (collection of melanin or skin pigment). These can be treated with laser also.

SKIN REJUVENATION

When we talk about ageing, skin is the first to be affected. Wrinkling, sagging, bags under eyes are natural consequences of ageing. A robust constitution, moderate exercise, good nutrition, adequate sleep and proper management of stress help in slowing down the process, but some artificial aids are also available for those of you who can afford them.

Now it is possible up to an extent to *reverse* the effects of aging on the skin by various methods. Some of these are discussed below.

a) **Dermabrasion**

Here the superficial skin layer is abraded so that new skin can grow. Our grandmothers used oatmeal, coarsely ground wheat or pulse powders mixed with various ingredients as scrubs. Now of course, we have advanced from sand paper to chemical peels, to the latest *electrical dermabrasion and laser,* giving good results.

b) **Face lifting**

Here electric current of low intensity is used to stimulate muscles of the face, thus toning them and 'lifting' the face from its sagging or wrinkled state Laser can also be used for this.

Surgical face lifting involves making an incision along the hairline and behind the ears, removing the flap of facial skin, cutting off the adherent bands under it, so that the skin can be stretched, to remove crows feet, wrinkles, and double chins, but remember, general anaesthesia (with its risks) has to be given and under inexpert hands your search for a youthful face may turn into a horror story.

Injectables and Skin Fillers

Injectable skin fillers have added new dimensions to the field of cosmetic dermatology, allowing new forms of facial rejuvenation and wrinkle treatment without surgery.

+ Polymethylmethacrylate (PMMA) microspheres suspended in bovine collagen

+ This injectable gives long lasting effect as it is not absorbed by the body unlike other fillers.

+ Botox-Botulinum toxin injection removes wrinkles by relaxing the facial muscles, but its action wears off in 3-6 months and has to be repeated. And if overdone it can lead to a mask like expressionless face.

+ Hyaluronic acid—removes wrinkles and smoothens skin, by absorbing water. But it can have temporary allergic reaction in some people.

+ Collagen injections can be derived from animals or humans and increases elastic tone of face.

+ Fascian—is made from fascia, a tissue from human body. It is thicker than normal collagen and effect lasts longer.

+ Fat injection—microlipoinjection is a procedure in which the doctor draws fat from the same patient's thighs or buttocks and injects it into the face. The effect can last for several years.

+ Micro spheres of calcium and phosphate ions--- this injection gives long lasting effect—removes wrinkles and smoothens skin.

+ Poly-L-Lactic Acid (PLLA) is diluted in sterile water and injected beneath skin to give volume and remove wrinkles.

REJUVENATING CREAMS

Look out for creams containing following ingredients and use them at night for maximal benefit. Those with oily skins should choose a formulation in gel or serum form.

Retinol or retino-A

use only at night as during day time it may burn the skin. It boosts collagen and elasten and gives a more youthful look.

Keratins

stimulate new skin growth, reduces wrinkles and inflammation.

Citric and Glycolic Acids

remove dead cells, and stimulate growth of new ones.

Squalene and Co-Q

revitalise skin

Hyaluronic Acid

'plumps up' skin and hides wrinkles.

Hydroquinone, Arbutin and Kojic Extracts

lighten dark pigmentation.

Aloevera, Jojoba extracts and Glycerine-

increase new cell formation.

Alpha and B-hydroxy Acids-

remove dead cells.

Peptides-

stimulate collagen production

EXERCISES TO PREVENT WRINKLES AND SAGGING

Fill up your cheeks with air or water, and hold as long as possible, and then blow it out very slowly. Next, open your eyes wide & maintain as long as you can. Repeat both exercises, five times. Alternatively fill up your mouth with water and hold as long as possible and splash cold water on your face as often as possible or just blow balloons (it will tone up your lungs and also please some kids!) These exercises, will retard the process of ageing, & add glow to the face.

FEW BASIC RULES

Finally a few basic rules to follow

1. Cleanse your skin twice a day

2. Treat the skin according to its type

3. Avoid excessive exposure to sunlight

4. Avoid oily, spicy food

5. Massage the body at least once a week

6. Avoid smoking

7. Eat nutritious food

8. Drink 8 glasses of water (2 liters a day)

9. Exercise regularly

10. Avoid late night activities and ensure adequate sleep.

✦✦✦✦

10

Imbalance, Insomnia & Headache

A) IMBALANCE

Next to headache and acidity, giddiness or imbalance is the commonest complaint of patients. Giddiness can be due to various causes such as indigestion or acidity, which can give us a feeling of 'black out', cervical spondylitis, as spine is involved in maintaining balance, or due to ear problems since ears also help to maintain equilibrium. Giddiness can also be due to fluctuations in blood pressure as both high and low pressure can lead to a feeling of imbalance. Similarly, fluctuations in blood sugar (both high and low) can lead to this feeling, although it is normally a sign of low blood sugar.

Sometimes eye problems can lead to giddiness or a feeling of imbalance, as eyes are needed for coordinated movements. Rarely the problem may be in the brain, or due to block in blood vessels, and lastly, it may be a sign of underlying mental depression. After finding out the cause, medication should be started. But any medication for idiopathic giddiness (where a cause is not found) should not be continued beyond 6 weeks, as the body's ability to adapt will suffer.

There are very good exercises for these patients which give good results if performed regularly (given below), these are adaptogenic exercises and can be done by normal people also, to strengthen their organs of balance. Hope you find them useful.

Adaptation Exercises For Giddiness And Vertigo

1) Eye Movements

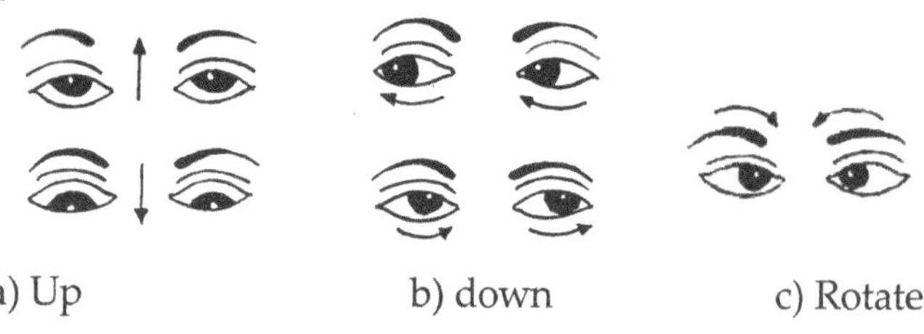

a) Up   b) down   c) Rotate

2) Neck Movements

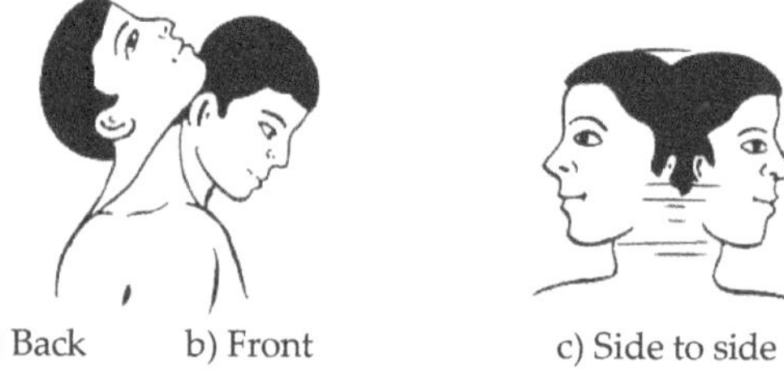

a) Back   b) Front   c) Side to side

3) While Sitting

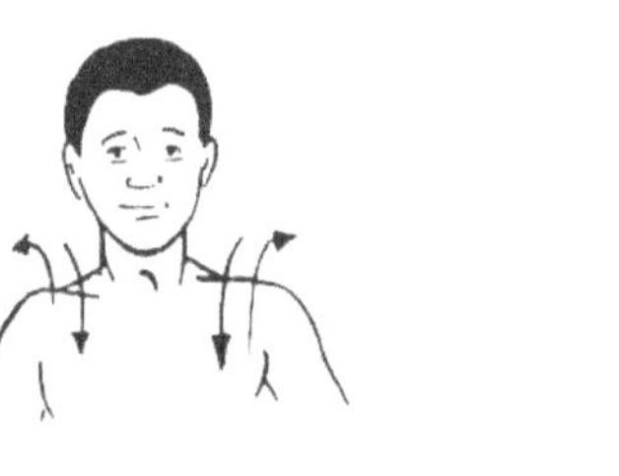

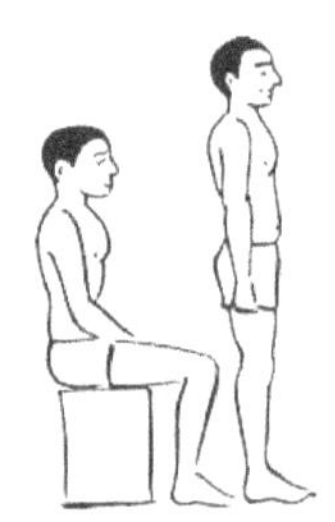

Shoulder rotation   Stand up & sit down

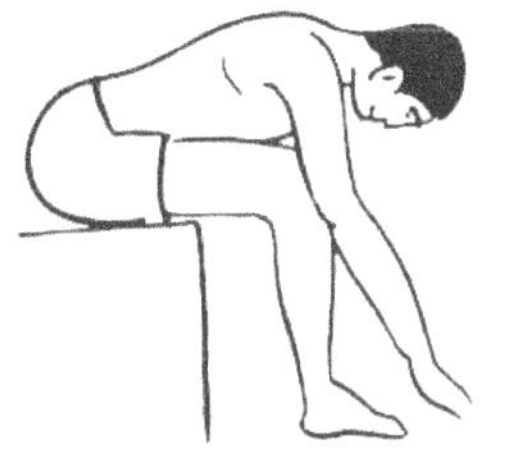

Bend down & move hands
from side to side.

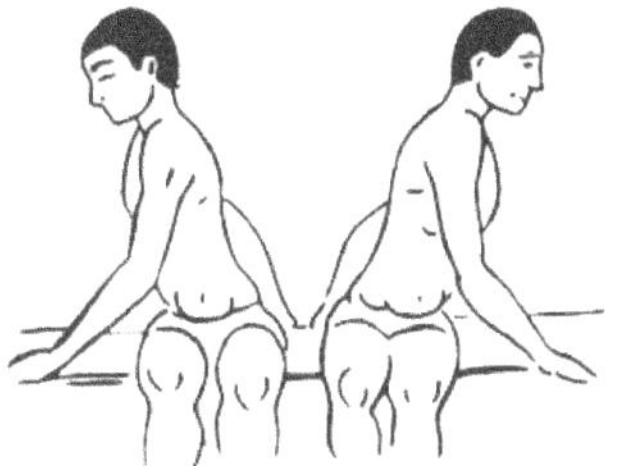

While sitting turn from
one side to the other

4) WHILE STANDING

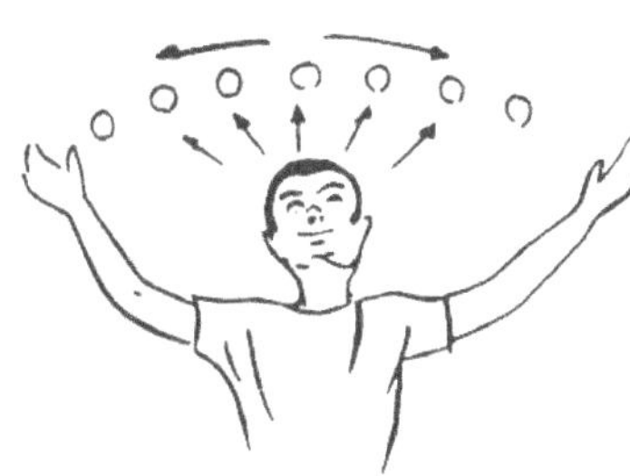

Throw ball from one hand to the
other looking up

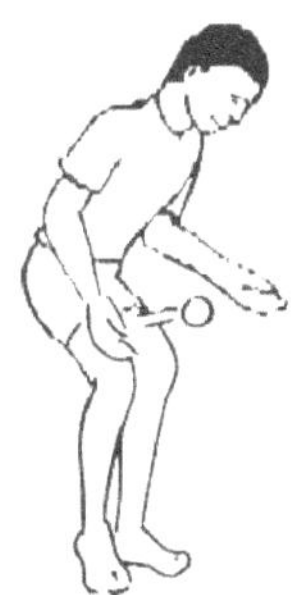

Reach up for ball and
then reach down

5) WHILE WALKING

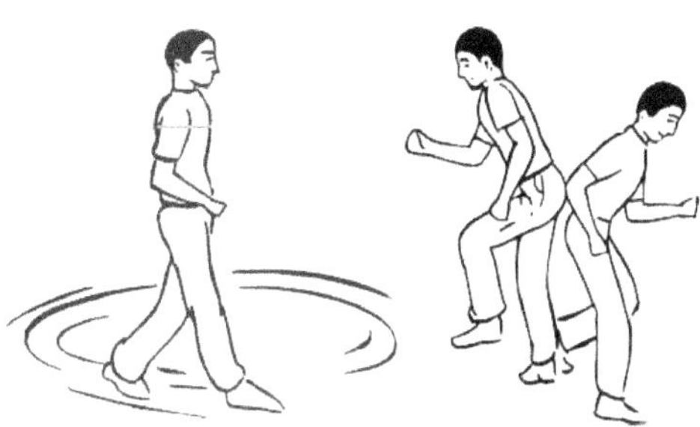

Walk in a circle

Walk up
down the stairs

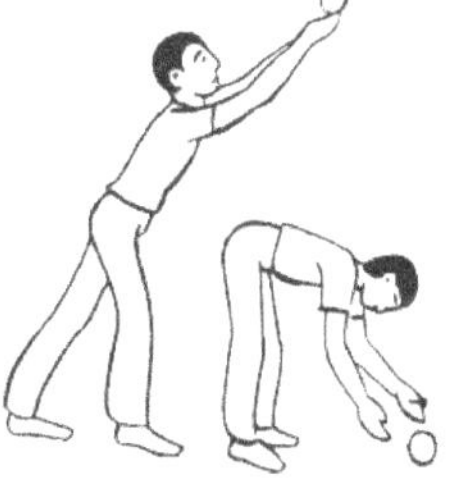

Reach up for ball and
then reach down

CHECKLIST OF CAUSES OF GIDDINESS:

1. Ears
2. Eyes
3. Neck
4. Acidity and indigestion
5. High or low blood pressure
6. Low blood glucose
7. Causes in brain and its blood vessels
8. Mental depression

B) INSOMNIA   (Sleeplessness)

What is normal sleep and how much of it does an average person need? Jawaharlal Nehru (former Indian prime minister) could make do with five hours of sleep at night, and Kumbhakarna a mythological figure, needed six months at a stretch! When a motor vehicle has been running for some time, it has to be overhauled at a garage, to clean and mend any faults, so that it can continue to function smoothly. Similarly when we sleep, our batteries are recharged, important repair work is carried out, and poisons and toxins cleared from the system, so that the next day, we can work more efficiently. Dreams are also a part of this cleansing mechanism, as the problems not solved during the day, surface at night, and the body attempts to deal with them so that they stop bothering us the next day.

On an average, seven to eight hours of sleep are enough in a healthy adult, and anything less than four hours or more than nine hours is known to reduce our life span. Sleep alternates between REM (rapid eye movement or dreaming sleep), and NREM or (non rapid eye movement) sleep.

Our nights begin with NREM sleep which lasts for 45–60 minutes goes on to REM sleep in 80 minutes and then this goes on throughout the night in alternate cycles of 90 to 110 minutes.

In REM sleep, blood pressure and heart rate become irregular and breathing muscles become lax, so chances of heart attacks and disturbed breathing are more. Thyroid and adrenal gland secretions, which control our metabolic rate and reaction to emergencies, also reduce and we are prone to the ill effects of temperature fluctuations.

I am sure robbers have made a deep study of sleep patterns, because they always strike when we are in REM sleep!

Causes of Insomnia

Insomnia could be due to numerous causes. The common ones are:

1. Physical stimuli like bright lights (even a luminous clock), external sounds, a snoring bed partner, extremes of temperatures, humming mosquitoes, an uncomfortable bed, unpleasant smells etc.

2. Pain: The next common cause of sleeplessness is pain. This can be pain in neck, head, cardiac (heart), pain of hyperacidity, general body ache, leg cramps etc.

3. Obstructed breathing - anything which causes 'choking up' or obstruction in breathing like snoring, a blocked nose or asthma can all lead to loss of sleep.

4. Frequent awakening to pass urine – due to diabetes, enlarged prostate gland or infection.

5. Anything, which causes a change in sleep rhythm like jet lag, shift duty etc.

6. Fasting or feasting – stomach should be neither empty nor uncomfortably full, to ensure a good night's sleep.

7. Drugs and addictions – drugs can cause sleeplessness like ephedrine, amphetamine, acute withdrawal of hypnotic drugs etc. Addictions like nicotine (smoking), alcohol and too much coffee can also interfere with sleep.

8. Emotional stress: It definitely interferes with normal sleep like exam tension, a tragic event etc.

9. Psychiatric disorders - Patients with psychiatric disorders have sleep problems, either too little or too much.

Management

Depending on the cause, insomnia should be managed, but there are a few guidelines:

1. Cut down on daytime sleep.

2. Increase physical activity – when we are tired out, chances of dropping off to sleep are more

3. Take a light but adequate dinner

4. A glass of milk at night was supposed to be grandma's remedy for a relaxed night. As usual she was right. Milk contains tryptophane, a natural sedative.

5. Oil massage on the head is also supposed to give sound sleep.

6. Avoid smoking, alcohol, coffee, chocolates, chocolate beverages or colas before going to bed.

7. Take care of any pains (acidity, heart pain, and body ache) before retiring.

8. If prone to night attacks of asthma – take an effective dose before going to bed.

9. Maintain regularity in sleeping time and uniformity in sleeping atmosphere.

10. Avoid stressful situations before going to bed.

11. Reading is a very good sleep inducer, but make sure your glasses are good and there is enough lighting.

12. Soft music, 'shavasana'(a yoga pose), and meditation also help

13. There is a gland in the brain called pineal gland, which

sets the body clock by secreting a substance called *melatonin*, which helps us to appreciate darkness, and induces sleep. Melatonin is now available commercially and helpful in inducing sleep especially in patients who do shift duty or have jet lag.

14. Even if you don't get sleep, relax, do some reading or mental work and you will find yourself dozing off.

15. Drugs should be resorted to only as a last resort, and for short courses under medical supervision as they can be addictive.

SNORING

Normally the air passages from the nose to the throat are clear and patent, and there is no obstruction to the flow of air. But when we sleep, the muscles of these passages are relaxed leading to their narrowing, which is further accentuated when we sleep on our back, as the tongue tends to fall back increasing the obstruction. Vibrations caused by air flowing through the obstructed passages bring about the typical sounds, which we call snoring. Inflammation of the passages due to colds and asthma or mechanical obstruction due to any cause will add to the problem. In 10-15% of cases, this obstructed breathing can lead to deficiency of oxygen or even a condition called *sleep apnoea* (a temporary state where air flow is totally cut off to the lungs.) These patients need to be seen by a specialist since some of the attacks can even prove life threatening.

Causes of Snoring

1. Being overweight.

2. Drinking alcohol at night.

3. Taking sedatives or tranquilisers.

4. Smoking.

5. Family history of snoring.

6. Short thick neck or a double chin.

7. Mechanical obstruction (growth or foreign body).

8. Hypothyroid state (low level of thyroid hormone).

9. Intake of drugs like-aspirin, female hormones, blood pressure medicines etc.

MANAGEMENT

1. Prevent the patient from sleeping on his back by tying something to the back like balls.

2. Avoid or cure any precipitating cause--obesity, drugs, diseases, smoking, alcohol etc.

3. Surgical resection of any obstruction

4. Various devices to keep the chin up and mouth closed.

5. CPAP (continuous positive pressure respiration)

   -a contraption, which ensures air entry under pressure to avoid sleep apnoea. It is not a very comfortable appliance and only those patients with severe obstruction will agree to wear it while sleeping. There are sleep clinics, which can identify the high-risk cases and also guide in management.

C) HEADACHE

"All that aches (in the head} may not be migraine!"

Headache can be due to numerous reasons, so remember - it may be dangerous to take an aspirin for it without knowing the cause. Aspirin should not be taken if there is bleeding or tendency towards bleeding from any part of the body or if a patient has hyperacidity, both these conditions as you will see can also cause headache. And it should be avoided in children less than 14 years of age since it can cause a condition called *Reye's syndrome* which can also be fatal.

The commonest cause of headache is of course *migraine.* Here, the blood vessels are more sensitive to certain chemicals from our body, and over-react to them, leading to first narrowing and then expansion. It is this second stage, in which we experience headache. In the first stage, we may feel faint, or uneasy, or have flashes of light in front of our eyes. - this is a warning of impending attack, and if we are driving a vehicle, we should immediately get off the road and take our medication, as it can be dangerous to drive during an attack. Other causes of headache may be from the stomach, face, ears, teeth, neck, eyes, muscles, arteries, nerves etc.

If there is hyperacidity, or if the *stomach* has remained empty for long or there is indigestion or constipation, we can have a dull headache.

High blood pressure and low blood sugar also can cause headache – so look out for these common causes.

Problems from the *face* like eyes, sinuses, ears, teeth, muscles, nerves and arteries - can all cause headaches as the same set of nerves supply the head and face. Hangover after an alcoholic binge the previous night can also cause headache.

Headache can also originate from the *neck* – from muscles or bones but the most serious causes of headache are from the *head* itself. These can be due to bleeding, as a result of rupture of blood vessels (due to high blood pressure or accidents) or to certain bleeding disorders. They can also be due to tumours, which may be malignant (cancerous) or benign (non-cancerous). Any new onset of headache or change in frequency, severity or character should make us suspect these serious causes. Headache can occasionally be due to certain forms of infections in the brain, and lastly it may be due to underlying *mental problems.* So next time you have a headache, think twice before popping an aspirin.

Management of Headache

It should be according to the cause. If no cause is found or it is migrainous, there are some good preventive drugs available. Discuss these with your doctor.

Diet: Avoid over-eating, under eating, sour and fermented foods, caffeine (coffee, soft drinks, chocolates, chocolate beverages), aging cheese (contains tyramine which is a powerful trigger for migraine). Take *magnesium*-containing foods (nuts, sprouts, beans, bananas, Soya and green leafy vegetables) as they influence blood vessel expansion, thus preventing migraine.

Other measures – Yoga, meditation, optimal sleep, stress management, exercise, massage, acupressure, and acupuncture are also helpful.

Management of Hadache

D - Diet, drugs

R - Relaxation techniques

E - Exercise

A - Acupressure, acupuncture

M - Massage

S - Sleep in adequate amounts

✦✦✦✦

Part – II

Problems
which can affect
Many of us

11

Management of Obesity

"The best e/ercise is to push yourself away from the dining table three times a day."

Gone are the days when plump bodies and chubby cheeks were considered cute, and a pot -belly was a status symbol to be flaunted along with flashy jewelry. Thin and trim is in today, but being thin is not only for the obvious cosmetic advantage, but mainly to avoid all the medical problems caused by obesity. Firstly, life expectancy of an overweight person is less than their

RISKS OF OBESITY

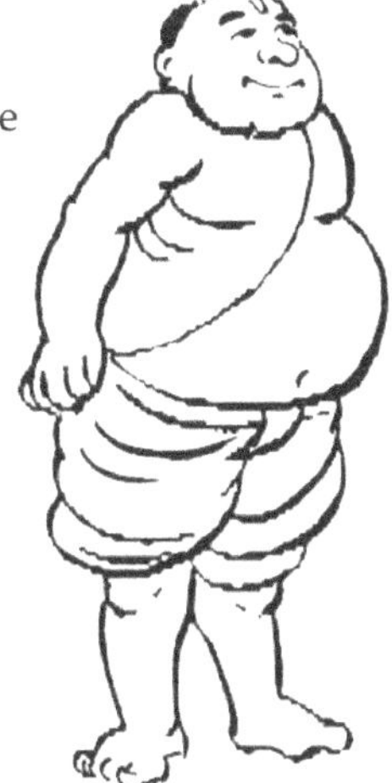

trimmer counterparts, and they are also susceptible to diabetes, blood pressure (especially if the person is 'pear-shaped' – that is, carries more girth around his/her tummy); as also arthritis, varicose veins (explained below), spondylitis, hernias, uterine prolapse, and delayed wound healing. Operating on, transporting, and handling an obese patient is also very difficult

VARICOSE VEINS

A very common problem after forty, especially in overweight women is that of *varicose-veins*. Here the veins become convoluted, prominent and visible. Since our legs are the furthest from the heart, it takes more effort to push the blood back into it through the leg veins. This is normally done by our leg muscles, which act like a pump. In obese people, there is deposition of fat between the muscle layers and so the pump becomes weak. As blood cannot be pushed up easily, it stagnates, leading to pain and swelling. There are also some valves in our leg veins, which allow only upward flow of blood. If the pump is weak, these valves break and there is further stagnation and tortuosity (twisting) of the veins to accommodate the extra blood. Women have been burdened with less muscles and extra fat for procreation, but it is up to them to build up their muscle mass so that there is efficient pumping action. Elastic (cotton) support stockings of good quality help in preventing stagnation of blood and certain medicines and a surgical or laser procedure called 'stripping' can also be performed. Some calf strengthening exercises to prevent and ameliorate (relieve) varicose veins have been included, among the exercises, in chapter 8.

Now that we have understood *why* we must lose weight, let us try to understand *how* we can do it. Being over weight is due to wrong habits developed early in life. Habits cannot be suddenly changed as Mark Twain has said; they have to be coaxed down the stairs one at a time. Remember, little drops of water make a mighty ocean and conversely *loss* of little drops at a time can change an ocean back into a river. So take it - a step at a time, a drop at a time, and don't cheat yourselves (I eat so little, and still I get fat!).

Obesity can be controlled by a combination of four methods-

a) Diet

b) Exercise

c) Behavioral and

d) Artificial methods

Now let us take them one by one-

DIET

Counting calories and weighted diets are cumbersome and hard to sustain. A diet should be easy to follow and built around a person's natural eating habits for it to be effective on a long-term basis. Ideally an overweight person should eat small, frequent meals, drink plenty of water and unsweetened drinks, reduce non-vegetarian food (too much protein and fat, too little fibre), avoid fried foods and conserve sugar and salt. They should be liberal with their intake of fibre- rich foods - like whole meal chapattis, brown bread, plenty of fruits and vegetables, sprouts, and spices - like black pepper, ginger, turmeric and fenugreek which help in burning fat and reducing lipids in blood. Incidentally there is a chemical called *leptin* in the body which helps in weight reduction by burning fat, and is also present in the poor mans food --whole roasted Bengal gram, especially in the covering, which is usually thrown away. A new kind of fat has also been discovered called, *orlistat* which is not absorbed, so you can eat your chips & not put on weight too! The only problem is that it can cause diarrhoea.

You must dilute every thing you take   -*To be thin, take thin!*

EXERCISE

After diet, comes exercise. Exercise, not only helps in reducing weight, it also tones up our system. Exercise can be aerobic (where the heart rate becomes fast and we perspire mildly) or anaerobic where more stress is laid on stretching and toning up of the body.

Examples of *Aerobic elercises* are - step exercises with music, brisk walking, jogging, skipping, swimming and fast games like badminton, tennis, squash and basketball.

Anaerobic elercises may be yoga, or weight training. Yoga tones up all the organs and systems, besides compressing our bodies into shape (like compressing a loose new cotton pillow into a tight one). We should combine aerobic and anaerobic exercises for best results.

Some Exercises For A Trim Abdomen

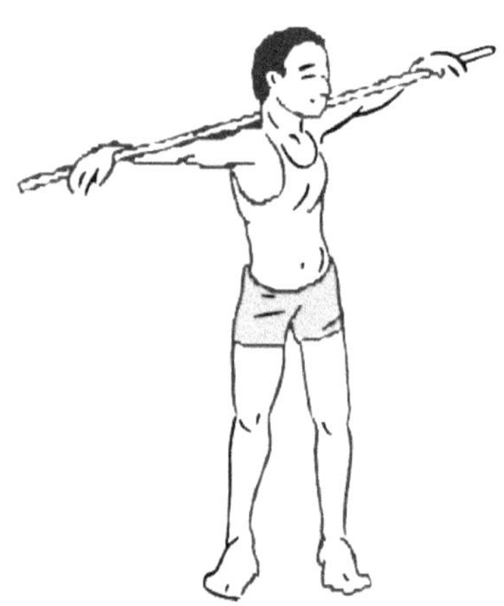

Stand with feet wide apart, holding a long stick behind the neck. Twist the upper body from side to side slowly keeping lower part of body still. Continue for 1-3 mts.

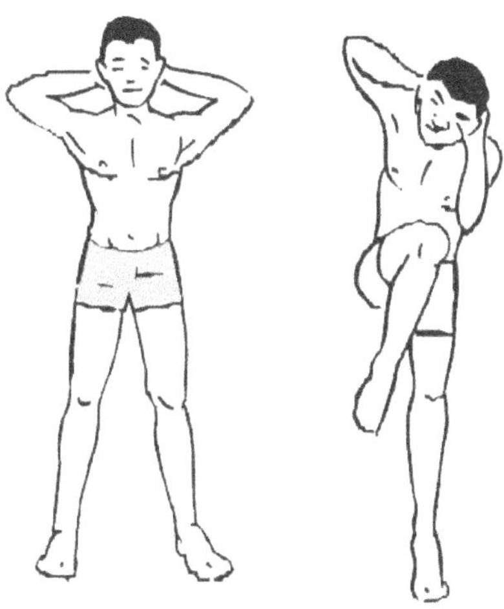

Stand as shown with your hands behind your neck, and lower
your left elbow to your right knee as you bring the knee up to
meet it. After returning to starting position repeat with right
elbow and left knee and keep repeating alternately moving as
smoothly as possible.

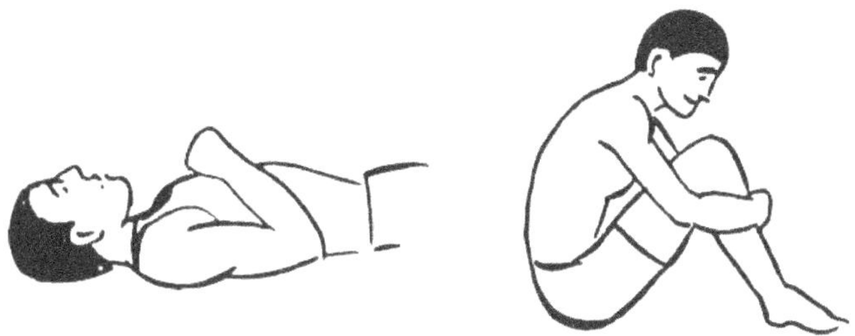

Lie on back with knees bent and feet flat on the floor. Now sit up
slowly first raising your head then your neck, then each vertebra
slowly as if peeling them one by one off the floor and move the
arms forward past the shins. Now slowly lie down again to the
original position. Keep repeating smoothly 10-15 times.

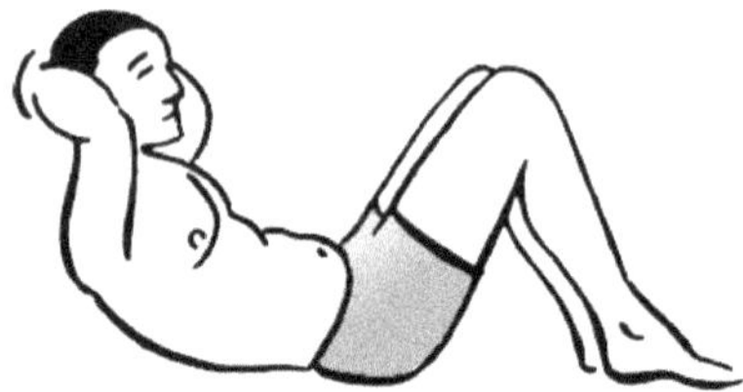

Lie on back with knees and feet flat on the floor and place
hands behind head elbows outwards pressing lower back on
floor. Now bend legs at knees, lift shoulders about three inches
from the floor keep looking towards the ceiling and slowly
lower them back. Repeat 10-15 times.

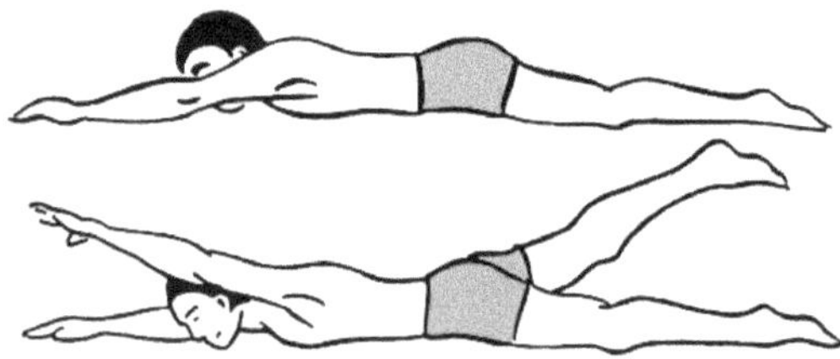

Lie on stomach with legs and arms extended, raise your right
leg and left arm, off the floor at the same time and slowly
lower Repeat 10-15times,then do the same with the left leg
and right arm

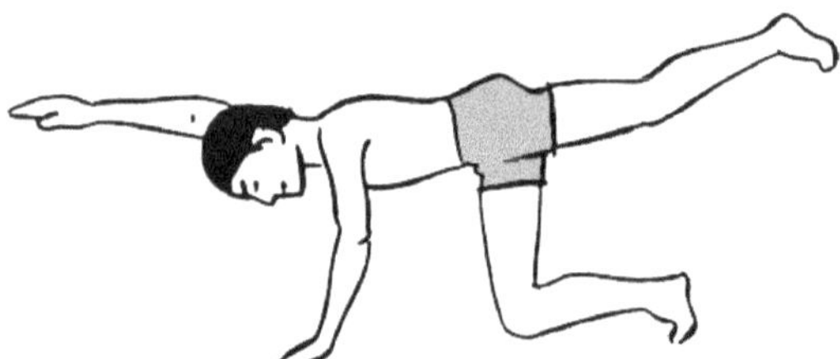

Kneel so that your neck is in line with your spine and
simultaneously raise your left hand and right leg tighten your
stomach and hold till a count of three. After returning to
kneeling position, repeat on opposite side alternating
10-15 times.

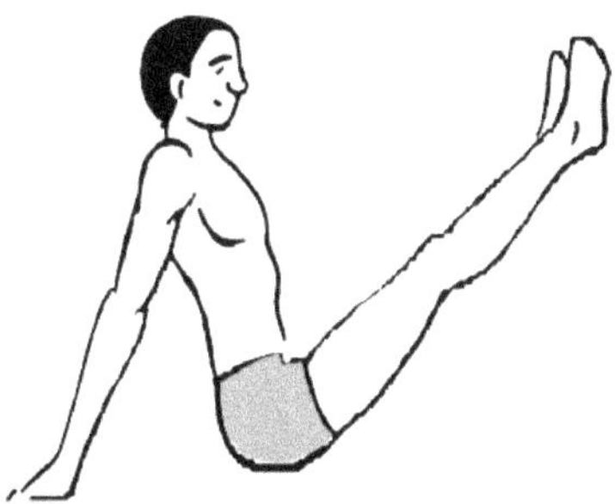

Sit comfortably on the floor with torso erect and hands extended behind you on either side. Keeping knees straight, raise legs as high as you can keeping body on floor. As you become fitter you can do this with your legs straightened at the knees (as shown).
Repeat 10- 15 times

Now here are some charts showing ideal body weight (IBW) and other parameters, weight watchers need to know about. See where you are placed.

Standard Height & Weight For Indian Men & Women

Height		Weight (Men)	Weight (Women)
Metre	Inches	Kg	Kg
1.52	5'-0"	–	50-54
1.54	5'-1"	–	51-55
1.57	5'-2"	56-60	53-56
1.59	5'-3"	57-61	54-58
1.62	5'-4"	59-63	56-60
1.65	5'-5"	61-65	58-61
1.67	5'-6"	62-67	59-64
1.70	5'-7"	64-68	61-65
1.72	5'-8"	66-71	62-67
1.75	5'-9"	68-73	64-69
1.77	5'-10"	69-74	66-70
1.80	5'-11"	71-76	67-72
1.82	6'-0"	73-78	69-74
1.85	6'-1"	75-81	-
1.87	6'-2"	77-84	-

Source: Life Insurance Corporation of India

BODY MASS INDEX

The Body Mass Index or B M I is a good index of obesity. It is calculated by dividing body weight in kilograms by height in metres squared.

	Good	Normal	Increased
Males	below 25	25-27	above 27
Females	below 23	23-25	above 25

Less than 25 - normal,   25 - 30 - is over weight More than 30 - is obese

BODY MASS INDEX - Ready Reckoner

Weight (Kg)	Height (cm)									
	145	150	155	160	165	170	175	180	185	190
50	24	22	21	20	18	17	16	15	15	14
52	25	23	22	20	19	18	17	16	15	14
54	26	24	22	21	20	19	18	17	16	15
56	27	25	23	22	21	19	18	17	16	16
58	28	26	24	23	21	20	19	18	17	16
60	29	27	25	23	22	21	20	19	18	17
62	29	28	26	24	23	21	20	19	18	17
64	30	28	27	25	24	22	21	20	19	18
66	31	29	27	26	24	23	22	20	19	18
68	32	30	28	27	25	24	22	21	20	19
70	33	31	29	27	26	24	23	22	20	19
72	34	32	30	28	26	25	24	22	21	20
74	35	33	31	29	27	26	24	23	22	20
76	36	34	32	30	28	26	25	23	22	21
78	37	35	32	30	29	27	25	24	23	22
80	38	36	33	31	29	28	26	25	23	22
82	39	36	34	32	30	28	27	25	24	23
84	40	37	35	33	31	29	27	26	25	23
86	41	38	36	34	32	30	28	27	25	24
88	42	39	37	34	32	30	29	27	26	24
90	43	40	37	35	33	31	29	28	26	25

if your height is 160 cms and weight is 68 kgs. your BMI is 27

WAIST HIP RATIO

Another important measurement is waist hip ratio. I already mentioned that increased girth around the waist is bad.

Waist circumference in centimeters divided by hip circumference in centimeters = W H R

WAIST HIP RATIO WAIST MEASURMENT (cms.) Ready Reckoner

50	55	60	65	70	75	(80)	85	90	95	100	105	110	115	120	125	130	135	140	.
1.00	1.10	1.20	1.30	1.40	1.50	1.60	1.70	1.80	1.90	2.00	2.10	2.20	2.30	2.40	2.50	2.60	2.70	2.80	50
0.91	1.00	1.09	1.18	1.27	1.36	1.45	1.55	1.64	1.73	1.82	1.91	2.00	2.09	2.18	2.27	2.36	2.45	2.55	55
0.83	0.92	1.00	1.08	1.17	1.25	1.33	1.42	1.50	1.58	1.67	1.75	1.83	1.92	2.00	2.08	2.17	2.25	2.33	60
0.77	0.85	0.92	1.00	1.08	1.15	1.23	1.31	1.38	1.46	1.54	1.62	1.69	1.77	1.85	1.92	2.00	2.08	2.15	65
0.71	0.79	0.86	0.93	1.00	1.07	1.14	1.21	1.29	1.36	1.43	1.50	1.57	1.67	1.71	1.79	1.86	1.93	2.00	70
0.67	0.73	0.80	0.87	0.93	1.00	1.07	1.13	1.20	1.27	1.33	1.40	1.47	1.53	1.60	1.67	1.73	1.80	1.87	75
0.63	0.69	0.75	0.81	0.88	0.94	1.00	1.06	1.13	1.19	1.25	1.31	1.38	1.44	1.50	1.56	1.63	1.69	1.75	80
0.59	0.65	0.71	0.76	0.82	0.88	0.94	1.00	1.06	1.12	1.18	1.24	1.29	1.35	1.41	1.47	1.53	1.59	1.65	85
0.56	0.61	0.67	0.72	0.87	0.83	(0.89)	0.94	1.00	1.06	1.11	1.17	1.22	1.28	1.33	1.39	1.44	1.50	1.56	(90)
0.53	0.58	0.63	0.68	0.74	0.79	0.84	0.89	0.95	1.00	1.05	1.11	1.16	1.21	1.26	1.32	1.37	1.42	1.47	95
0.50	0.55	0.60	0.65	0.70	0.75	0.80	0.85	0.90	0.95	1.00	1.05	1.10	1.15	1.20	1.25	1.30	1.35	1.40	100
0.48	0.52	0.57	0.62	0.67	0.71	0.76	0.81	0.86	0.90	0.95	1.00	1.05	1.10	1.14	1.19	1.24	1.29	1.33	105
0.45	0.50	0.55	0.59	0.64	0.68	0.73	0.77	0.82	0.86	0.91	0.95	1.00	1.05	1.09	1.14	1.18	1.23	1.27	110
0.43	0.48	0.52	0.57	0.61	0.65	0.70	0.74	0.78	0.83	0.87	0.91	0.96	1.00	1.04	1.09	1.13	1.17	1.22	115
0.42	0.46	0.50	0.54	0.58	0.63	0.67	0.71	0.75	0.79	0.83	0.88	0.92	0.96	1.00	1.04	1.08	1.13	1.17	120
0.40	0.44	0.48	0.52	0.56	0.60	0.64	0.68	0.72	0.76	0.80	0.84	0.88	0.92	0.96	1.00	1.04	1.08	1.12	125
0.38	0.42	0.46	0.50	0.54	0.58	0.62	0.65	0.69	0.73	0.77	0.81	0.85	0.88	0.92	0.96	1.00	1.04	1.08	130
0.37	0.41	0.44	0.48	0.52	0.56	0.59	0.63	0.67	0.70	0.74	0.78	0.81	0.85	0.89	0.93	0.96	1.00	1.04	135
0.36	0.39	0.43	0.46	0.50	0.54	0.57	0.61	0.64	0.68	0.71	0.75	0.79	0.82	0.88	0.89	0.93	0.96	1.00	140
0.34	0.38	0.41	0.45	0.48	0.52	0.55	0.59	0.62	0.68	0.69	0.72	0.76	0.79	0.83	0.86	0.90	0.93	0.97	145
0.33	0.37	0.40	0.43	0.47	0.50	0.53	0.57	0.60	0.63	0.67	0.70	0.73	0.77	0.80	0.83	0.87	0.90	0.93	150

Hip Measurement cms

WHR More than 0.95- is abdominal obesity in males
More than 0.85- is abdominal obesity in females

We should try to keep our I B W, B M I and W H R within the normal range to remain healthy.

W H R

| More than 0.95 | - is abdominal obesity in males |
| More than 0.85 | - is abdominal obesity in females |

$$\frac{\text{Waist circumference in centimetre}}{\text{Hip circumference in centimetre}} = WHR$$

We should try to keep our I B W, B M I and W H R within the normal range to remain healthy.

Now what is our caloric requirement?

Calorie is a measure of energy in food items (1 gm. of carbohydrate = 4 calories, 1 gram of fat = 9 calories, and 1 gm. of protein = 4.4 calories.) Calorie requirement of a person from various foods should be sufficient to maintain I B W (ideal body weight) over a prolonged time.

If we are over weight, we must consume	20 cal/kg/day
If we have I B W then	30 cal/kg/day
And if underweight then	40 cal/kg/day

We must add or subtract 5 – 10 cal/kg/day according to whether we are heavy or sedentary workers. A pregnant woman needs extra 500 cal/day and lactating woman 550cal/day additionally. We require 10% less than the total calories/day for our weight, for each decade after fifty years.

HOW TO CALCULATE YOUR CALORIC REQUIREMENT

Say, a man seventy years old, 170 centimeters tall of medium frame weighs 75 kgs. His I B W should be 63-65 kg. Therefore he needs 75 times 20 = 1500 calories/day. But since he is two decades above fifty years, he needs 20% less i.e. 1500 – 20% (300) = 1200 cal/day only. When computing our calorie requirement, we should also take into account the energy we expend in various activities (given below)

Energy that we burn during various activities is as under:

Walking

Walking slowly (2 MPH)	200 cal/hr
Walking briskly (5 MPH)	450 cal/hr
Jogging (5.5 MPH)	540 cal/hr
Running (7.2 MPH)	570 cal/hr
Walking uphill	1100 cal/hr

Exercise

Light exercise	170 cal/hr
Active exercise	290 cal/hr
Severe exercise	600 cal/hr
Very severe exercise	650 cal/hr

Games

Badminton	270 cal/hr
Golf	333 cal/hr
Tennis	450 cal/hr
Swimming/horse riding	500 cal/hr
Squash	630 cal/hr

Miscellaneous

Sewing (tailoring)	135 cal/hr
Typing rapidly	140 cal/hr
Dancing	273 cal /hr

Example - suppose our daily requirement of calories according to our height, body frame, age and moderate work habit is 1500 cal / day. Now if we walk uphill everyday for half an hour, we should add 550 calories to our daily requirement. Thus we need 1500 + 550 cal = 2050 calories/day (If we want to lose weight – we *don't* add these calories). *Burning 7700 K calories, leads to reduction in 1 kg of body weight.*

WALKING:

Walking is the best, cheapest and safest exercise we can perform at any age. We can walk in 10 minute spurts through- out the day or at a stretch. Generally fifteen kilometers of walking in a week is good enough to keep our body toned up *–So walk away from ill health!*

**"Take care of your inches and
your kilos wills take care of themselves"**

is another important adage to remember if we want to lose weight.

We should understand that there are three stages in losing weight—

    Stage 1— arrest of further gain.

    Stage 2— reduction in inches.

    Stage 3— actual reduction in weight.

So if you are on a weight reduction program, & find that your body is getting into shape, but the weighing scale, plays spoil sport, do not panic! It only means that your muscle-mass is increasing, and if you persist with your efforts, your weighing scale will start obeying your wishes, as fat loss from muscles, is much easier and faster.

FEW POINTS ABOUT JOGGING:

+ Wear light cotton clothing.

+ Wear track suit or another layer of clothing before & after jogging.

+ Wear light shoes with thick heels.

+ Wear thick cotton socks.

+ Don't jog within 2 hours of major meal.

Management of Obesity

+ Walk 5 minutes before & after jogging.

+ Heels should come down every time after toes.

+ Run on mud or grass to avoid strain to calves.

+ Relax shoulders & arms while jogging.

+ Distance covered &speed should be within limits of comfort.

+ If chest pains, or breathlessness develops, --STOP!

BEHAVIORAL METHODS FOR LOSING WEIGHT

(how the family can help)

Diet and exercise may not suffice for losing weight unless they are accompanied by behavioral changes. Let us understand some of these.

1. **Disturbance in body image of self**

   Overweight people especially those putting on weight at an early age, (when projecting a good image is very important,) can become so depressed with the (self perceived) negative image of themselves that they tend to avoid facing up to the fact that they are obese. This makes them particularly resistant to management. Here grooming and a little attention to looks if a female, and body building if a male accompanied by counseling are very helpful as they increase the feel-good factor and make them more cooperative in the endeavour to lose weight. They must also gently be made to understand that their type of obesity is more difficult to reverse, since the number of fat cells increase in childhood obesity, and we can only reduce their size and not their number while trying to reduce weight, and also sustained efforts may be required to maintain the weight later.

2.   **Availability of food**

Overweight people tend to eat more than normal people when more food is available to them and they also avoid putting in much effort to obtain food. Less food should therefore be available to them and preferably in an uncooked state or they should be encouraged to shop and cook for themselves. Availability of snacks especially should be totally checked, and those who cannot stop snacking, a good adage for them is — *if you can't avoid the snacks between the meals, avoid the meals between the snacks!*

3.   **Tasty food**

Obese individuals tend to eat more than non-obese when given tasty food, hence it is important to give them food, which is nutritious but not very tasty.

4.   **Time of eating**

if the time of eating can be progressively postponed by keeping them occupied with work or activity, they will tend to eat less.

5.   **Snacking**

Entertainment, partying and feasting even in the name of religion should be discouraged. Watching too much T.V also tends to make people sedentary and prone to snacking.

6.   **Group therapy**

They must join up with other overweight people to remind themselves that there are many people like them and also to compare notes, socialise, and help each other.

7.   **Movement**

Obese people are generally lazy and tend to get work done from others. They should be actively encouraged to do their own work (if not other's too!)

8. Also put this where they can read it everyday   -

"When I can sit,

I will not lie down

When I can stand

I will not sit

When I can walk,

I will not stand!   and

When I can run

I will not walk!"

ARTIFICIAL MEASURES

There are many artificial methods, of losing weight. Only those who are morbidly fat or cannot exercise should resort to these. Some of them are-

1. **Appetite suppressants-**

    a) **High fibre**

    b) **High protein powders** - they have been known to cause heart disease in USA.

    c) **Drugs** – like *sibutramine* (lowers appetite) and *orlistat* (reduces fat absorption by body) they should be taken only under medical supervision and only by those patients who have increased medical risks because of their obesity and not for cosmetic reasons. *Semaglutide* is a new anti Diabetic drug that also helps in weight reduction.

2. **Herbal preparations**

    Which "burn" fat. -Take them with caution.

Management of Obesity

3. **Liposuction** - to remove fat selectively from some areas-should be done only by very experienced cosmetic surgeons & in limited quantities only, so as not to endanger life.

4. **"Wiring"** of mouth (outdated!!!)

5. **Surgery** - Surgically reducing the size of stomach, to reduce food intake.

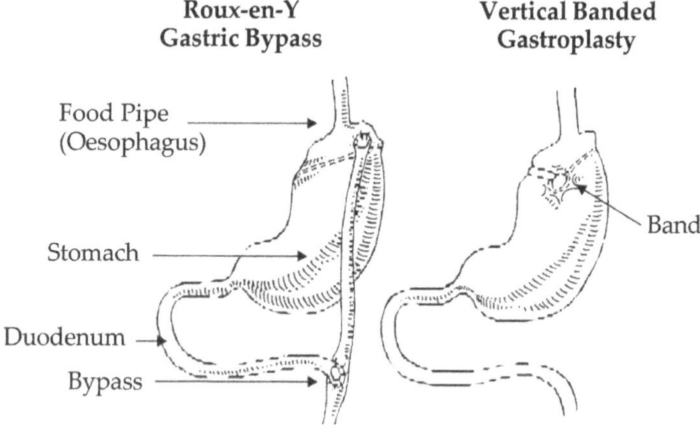

In **banded gastroplasty surgery**, the stomach size is reduced so that less food can be eaten, and in **Roux-en-Y surgery** besides reducing size of stomach, the duodenum is also bypassed,(which secretes many digestive juices),thus also reducing digestion. These surgeries are meant for those who are extremely obese and cannot exercise.

Reducing weight is possible if sufficient and sustained motivation is there. Combine anaerobic with some aerobic e/ercises, correct your diet, and you will soon see results, – remember a drop at a time is enough.

✦✦✦✦

12

Hypertension
- A Silent Killer

"Over-inflation is dangerous, in egos, tyres, &   blood vessels!"

The title of this chapter has been purposely chosen, as many people have no complaints when they have high blood pressure, and it remains 'silent' as it quietly goes about its job of destroying the body from within if left uncontrolled.

What is Hypertension?

The pressure exerted by the heart to pump blood into our blood vessels, is called blood pressure. Let us take the example of a cycle tube - the pressure in the tube can go up more than normal if there is a narrowing or choking up of the tube or some obstruction at the end, or if more air is pumped in, than the tube's capacity.

The story is the same in our arteries. Hypertension can occur because of increased *volume* of blood, *narrowing* of arteries or increase in the *peripheral resistance* to flow of blood back to the heart. Due to narrowing of arteries of limbs especially in the legs, the heart has to pump harder for the blood to reach the furthest parts, and because of this, over a period of time its size enlarges although pumping capacity reduces. As a consequence less blood goes to various organs especially kidneys, brain, heart, limbs and eyes, leading to a slow damage of all these organs and causing paralysis, heart attack, blindness, kidney failure and gangrene of limbs which may even require amputation. Sometimes these blood vessels in eyes, aorta (major artery) or brain may burst (because they cannot bear so much pressure and get thinned out after sometime) - causing brain haemorrhage (bleeding), bleeding inside the eyes (retinal haemorrhage), etc. Imagine all the changes due to blood pressure may be silently taking place in the body, and we may remain blissfully unaware, or more tragically, knowingly careless, since we know that we have blood pressure but choose to keep it untreated. 'Why should I get my blood pressure treated? I have no complaints,' is a common query from patients, and hopefully after reading this, a few of them will start taking regular medication.

What is Atherosclerosis?

Atheros means artery and sclerosis means hardening- so atherosclerosis means hardening of the blood vessels due to deposition of fats, followed by cells, sticky substances and finally calcium.

What is systolic and Diastolic Blood Pressure?

When the force of the pressure exerted by the heart is the greatest, it is called systolic blood pressure, and when the heart is relaxed, or exerting least pressure, what we measure is called diastolic blood pressure.

Normal Blood Pressure

There is no single level of pressure, which is "normal". But on an average anything from 100-140mm of mercury systolic or 60-90mm of mercury diastolic is considered normal. Blood pressure also increases with age. We have a formula, (for systolic blood pressure)

AGE +100 = Normal blood pressure, for your age. For example if you are forty years old, your systolic blood pressure, should not exceed 40+100, =140mmof mercury. But lately the tendency is to maintain a tighter control *at any age.* For example even in an eighty year old, we would not like to maintain 180 mm of mercury systolic blood pressure for long.

COMPLAINTS

Patients of hypertension may present with any of the following complaints - headache, palpitations (being conscious of one's heart beats), dizziness, flushed face, nose-bleed, breathlessness, blurred sight etc.

SECONDARY BLOOD PRESSURE

Normally blood pressure is called *primary* or *essential* blood pressure, which is not curable, but can only be kept under control. But there are certain diseases that can cause secondary blood pressure that may be curable.

These are called **Secondary Blood Pressures**.

They may be due to -

1.	Kidney diseases - A diseased kidney or a narrowing in a kidney blood vessel can cause hypertension, as kidneys are responsible for maintaining salt balance and they also secrete a chemical, which increases blood pressure.

2.	Certain Tumours - of glands in our abdomen (stomach) called "phaeochromocytoma" - can cause very high and fluctuating blood pressure.

3.	Increase in activity of another gland called adrenal gland can cause "Cushings disease" which can also cause high blood pressure.

4. Drugs- steroids, anti- inflammatory drugs, and contraceptive pills (birth control pills) can cause reversible high blood pressure.

Any of the above causes if treated can cure the high blood pressure.

PRECIPITATING CAUSES

Now what can increase our chances of getting high blood pressure? These may be-

1. Obesity
2. Smoking
3. Coffee
4. Stress
5. Alcohol
6. Family history of blood pressure
7. Lipid abnormality
8. Some drugs
9. Hyper-insulinaemia

Now let us consider these one by one -

1. **Obesity** - when we are over-weight, our heart has to pump blood to a greater body mass obviously increasing the "pressure" on our blood vessels.

2. **Smoking** - causes narrowing of vessels due to release of certain chemicals.

3. **Coffee** - excessive intake of coffee can also increase blood pressure probably by causing narrowing of vessels.

4. **Stress** - mental tension causes release of certain chemicals in the body which leads to narrowing of blood vessels and hence rise in blood pressure.

5. **Alcohol** - alcohol intake in moderation can cause rise in blood pressure. Additionally, snacking and feasting

leading to obesity usually accompany alcohol intake.

6. **Family history of blood pressure**-. If there is family history of blood pressure, tendency towards hypertension is more.

7. **Dyslipidaemia** - increase in bad fats and decrease in good fats hastens atherosclerosis and thus blood pressure.

8. **Drugs** - long-term intake of certain drugs, like steroids and anti- arthritic drugs can increase blood pressure.

9. **Hyper insulinaemia** - increased levels of insulin in the blood, can lead to obesity, hypertension & atherosclerosis.

DIET IN HYPERTENSION

Firstly let us consider –

SALT

there is no proof that increased intake of salt can increase our blood pressure, but if our pressure is already high, cutting down on salt helps. Our body actually requires only 2000 milligrams of salt in a day from food, which can increase in summer, but most of us consume 30-50 times that amount. Try to avoid highly salted and preserved foods like pickles and salted snacks. Normal salt contains 40% *sodium.* You can use low sodium salts available in the market, which contain only 18 % sodium. On the other hand *calcium, magnesium and potassium* keep the blood pressure low. Best source of potassium are fruits. Greens and dairy products supply enough calcium, and magnesium is present in nuts sprouts Soya beans and bananas.

Diet for hypertension should therefore be vegetarian (plus fish), high in fibre, a lot of fruits (they provide fibre and potassium), plenty of vegetables, avoidance of solid fats (ghee(clarified butter), butter, margarine, cheese), and less of refined foods like refined flour, sugar etc. Salt should be restricted and highly salted items like pickles, chutneys, and salted snacks should be strictly avoided.

DASH DIET (Dietary Approaches to Stop Hypertension)

This is a dietary pattern promoted by the U.S.-based National Heart, Lung, and Blood Institute (part of the National Institutes of Health, an agency of the United States Department of Health and Human Services) to prevent and control hypertension. The DASH diet is rich in fruits, vegetables, whole grains, and low-fat dairy foods; includes fish, poultry, nuts and beans; and is limited in sugar-sweetened foods and beverages, red meat, and added fats. In addition to its effect on blood pressure, it is considered a well-balanced approach to eating for the general public. It is now recommended by the US Department of Agriculture (USDA) as an ideal eating plan for all Americans

The US Dietary Guidelines for Americans recommend eating a diet of 2300 mg of sodium a day or lower, with a recommendation of 1500 mg/day in adults who have elevated blood pressure; the 1500 mg/day is the low sodium level tested in the DASH-Sodium study.

At sodium intake level of 1,500 mg/day, plus the other recommendations of DASH diet, there was an average blood pressure reduction of 8.9/4.5 mm Hg (systolic/diastolic). Hypertensive subjects experienced a higher average reduction of 11.5/5.7 mm Hg. This reduction in blood pressure is in fact equal to that achieved by a single anti hypertensive drug.

OTHER MEASURES

In all except the severe cases of newly diagnosed hypertension, a trial of life style modification, diet, exercise, yoga, meditation and weight reduction can be made before resorting to medication.

CASE STUDIES

Let me tell you about two of my patients. The first was a massive personality, a senior banker, who came to the clinic with the only complaint of feeling 'hot' and on examination his B.P. was 260/140 mm Hg. He insisted I give him only immediate treatment and refused admission, in spite of my strongly advising it. After half an hour, his blood pressure came down, he felt better and left in a hurry, as he had to catch a train. Since his was a transferable job, I did not see him again for the next ten years. After this, he came to see me, now very trim, and insisted I knew him. He then told me that he had come to apologise for disregarding my advice of taking regular medication as after a few months he suffered a massive heart attack. He had undergone bypass surgery and was rehabilitated. Luckily for him he survived and learnt his lesson.

The second case I want to discuss is that of a lady who came from a business family, and was severely hypertensive and overweight when I first saw her. She also had very high dyslipidaemia (increase of bad fats in blood), her eating habits were irregular, and exercise in any form was non-existent. Her early years had been very hard trying to make both ends meet while bringing up four daughters and a son, on the shoe string budget provided by her shopkeeper husband. She had also sewed clothes in her spare time to earn some extra money. When I told her to stop eating rich and fried foods, which she loved, her poignant reply was that when she was allowed to eat these things she could not afford them, and now that she could afford them, she was not being allowed to eat them! She also felt that she had worked very hard all her life and now she wanted to relax, and not be forced into any exercise regimen. She remained irregular with her intake of medicines too, and as expected one day suffered a paralytic attack. After she had recovered from this we thought that she would be more cooperative with us in our efforts to bring about a change in her lifestyle, but it was not to be. A few years later, she had a mild heart attack, followed by another massive one in my clinic itself. We worked hard to bring her around and succeeded too, but a few months later she had a paralytic attack on the other side of her body. Now for the first time she was really scared and became very obedient, but it was too late and she continued to slide downhill until one day we finally lost her. The idea of presenting this case in detail is to illustrate how complications like paralysis and heart attack can occur in uncontrolled hypertensives as in this case or blindness and kidney failure as in many others, and hopefully influence a few readers into changing their ways and taking care of their blood pressure properly so that complications can be avoided and a few lives saved.

There is a condition called *"white coat hypertension"* which may not require treatment. Here, the blood pressure shoots up only when the doctor examines, at other times being normal. If this is suspected, 24 hours ambulatory B.P. monitoring called *"holter monitoring"* can be conducted. This is done with a simple device attached to the patient who then continues his/her normal activities and B.P. through out the day is recorded.

B.P. is also supposed to fall at night when we sleep. In some patients this does not happen and they are called *"nocturnal non dippers"*. These patients are at a higher risk for complications and their blood pressure should be strictly kept under control. This condition can also be diagnosed by ambulatory monitoring.

Self Monitoring Devices:

of various types for measuring blood pressure are now available but they need to be checked for accuracy regularly by your doctor.

Low Blood Pressure?

A lot of patients complain of *low* blood pressure. Patients with complaints like weakness, giddiness etc. when accompanied by a reading of blood pressure below 120/80 mm Hg, are wrongly labeled as suffering from low blood pressure. Actually this level may be normal for them. It is important to understand that there is no such disease as "low blood pressure". Blood pressure can fall due to loss of blood (any cause of bleeding) or fluids (diarrhoea, vomiting) or severe illness. Here blood pressure has fallen and we correct it, but we do not say the patient is suffering from "low blood pressure". Many patients can get psyched into thinking that they have a serious illness by having this label put on them. It is therefore important to remove this myth from people's minds.

Resistant Hypertension

Resistant hypertension is a severe type of high blood pressure that's difficult to control, even with multiple medications. People, who develop this condition, are at higher than average risk for strokes, heart attacks, kidney disease, and heart failure. Resistant hypertension affects about 1 in 11 people who have high blood pressure. They're very thin, exercise regularly, eat right and are on four medications and it's still very difficult to control their blood pressure. There are two new methods of treatment for such people-

1. The first is a procedure that deactivates overactive nerves in the kidneys; the procedure is done under local anesthesia. Doctors make a small incision in an artery near the groin and use it to thread a catheter up to the kidneys. A machine then fires short bursts of radio waves to deaden the sympathetic nerves.

2. **In the second procedure-** scientists found that removing the grain-sized carotid body - one of the tiniest organs in the human body may treat high blood pressure. The carotid body is a small nodule (no larger than a rice

grain) found on the side of each carotid artery in the neck and appears to be a major culprit in the development and regulation of high blood pressure. Normally, the carotid body acts to regulate the amount of oxygen and carbon-dioxide in the blood. They are stimulated when oxygen levels fall in the blood as happens when you hold your breath. Stimulation of carotid bodies causes a dramatic increase in breathing and blood pressure until blood oxygen levels are restored. University of Bristol researchers found that by removing the carotid body connection to the brain in rodents with high blood pressure, blood pressure fell and remained low.

If you take care of your hypertension with regular monitoring and medication, there is no reason why you cannot enjoy the life style and life span of a non-hypertensive - so take heart!

✦✦✦✦

13

Diabetes

"CONTROL is the key word in emotions & passions, as in Diabetes."

Dhanwantari, the ancient Indian physician called Diabetes 'Madhumeha' or sweet urine. It is a disease of "starvation amidst plenty" where the blood is rich in sugar, but it cannot be utilised, *due to lack of insulin or a resistance to its action.* It is like being out at sea with water all around us, which cannot be drunk, or outside a locked granary full of grain with the keys (insulin) being lost. Diabetes can be hereditary or acquired. Hereditary diabetes normally manifests at an earlier age (before forty), is seen more in men or in women during pregnancy, whereas acquired diabetes is due to wrong life style or environmental causes. Thirty years back the incidence of diabetes was 2% in urban areas and now it is 12-16%. In fact after the age of fifty, every second Indian is either a diabetic or a pre-diabetic (one who will soon get diabetes)! You can see the worldwide *rate of increase* of Diabetes from the following table -

+ An estimated 285 million people, corresponding to 6.4% of the world's adult population, will live with diabetes in 2010. The number is expected to grow to 438 million by 2030, corresponding to 7.8% of the adult population.

+ While the global prevalence of diabetes is 6.4%, the prevalence varies from 10.2% in the Western Pacific to 3.8% in the African region. However, the African region is expected to experience the highest increase.

+ 70% of the current cases of diabetes occur in low- and middle income countries. With an estimated 50.8 million people living with diabetes, India has the world's largest diabetes population, followed by China with 43.2 million.

Sedentary life style with obesity, especially 'central obesity' (fat accumulating around the internal organs or viscera) is a common cause of diabetes and, there is a condition called 'hyper insulinaemia' where there is too much insulin but of no use to the patient as it cannot act. These patients normally have central obesity dyslipidaemia (increase in bad fats and decrease in good fat) and hypertension too. They are said to suffer from 'metabolic syndrome'. Any disease, where the pancreas gets destroyed, can also cause diabetes, since the pancreas secretes insulin. Sometimes, certain medications (like steroids) can precipitate diabetes - so be cautious about taking any long-term medication without proper medical supervision. Conversely, there are many medications, which you should not take if you are a diabetic, so always inform any new doctor about your diabetic status.

+ Diabetes can be insulin dependant Diabetes Mellitus—IDDM or type-I.

+ Non-insulin dependant -NIDDM OR TYPE-II.

  Insulin dependant diabetes usually occurs at an earlier age (before forty) and NIDDM after the age of forty.

+ There is a third type called MODY or maturity onset diabetes of young.

✦ There is a disease called "fibrocystic disease of the pancreas" where the pancreas gets destroyed in patients who are mal-nourished, and many thin diabetics after forty, have this acquired cause of diabetes. And another important type of diabetes is -

✦ LADA (Latent autoimmune diabetes in adults). LADA occurs in thin people after the age of forty and without other 'metabolic' features.LADA is important because these patients rapidly progress to insulin need after a few years of control with oral drugs. They therefore begin like type –II diabetes but rapidly progress to Type-I.

Before we go any further, let us understand clearly-

As of today, diabetes cannot be cured; it can only be controlled --- So if anybody tells you otherwise, take it with a pinch of salt.

Now let us see how diabetes presents itself:

There are a few common symptoms (complaints) by which we can detect diabetes - like polyuria (excessive urination), polydypsia (excessive thirst) and polyphagia (excessive hunger). Besides these – non- healing wounds, non-responding infections, recent loss of weight, or any complaint due to complications (involvement of eyes, heart, limbs, brain, blood vessels, kidneys, nerves etc.) can be the presenting feature.

Management

Management of diabetes comprises – Diet, exercise, weight reduction, care of body (especially feet), regular medication, regular monitoring, and regular follow-up.

There are a lot of myths and misinformation about diabetes – so don't get influenced by quacks and so called well wishers who may lead you entirely along the wrong path.

Like hypertension, diabetes is **a** *silent killer* if improperly managed. It can damage eyes, heart, brain, limbs, kidneys, blood vessels and nerves. Once these complications occur, it may be very difficult to reverse them unless they are detected early, so it is very important that we prevent them from occurring *by keeping our blood glucose under control.*

Diet

A diabetic should avoid both fasting and feasting. He/she should take small frequent four hourly meals, which will avoid a load on the pancreas. A thin diabetic can take more calories but change its quality; however an obese diabetic has to change both.

Simple sugars like sugar, unrefined sugar & honey should be totally avoided as also refined foods like refined flour, potatoes and white rice.

Sweet fruits like-bananas, mangoes, custard apple and grapes should be preferably avoided.

All these foods have a 'high glycaemic index', that is they cause sugar to rise rapidly in blood.

 Saturated fats should be cut down too – like ghee (clarified butter),butter, cheese and hydrogenated oils (margarine).Unsaturated oils should also be taken in moderation to avoid obesity. Non-vegetarian foods (being low in fibre and high in proteins and fats) should be avoided as far as possible except for fish, which is good.

Diabetics should take a fibre rich diet with plenty of vegetables, sprouts and less sweet fruits like citrus fruits, berries, pomegranate, papaya, grape-fruit etc. Chapattis and bread should be made from whole meal cereals. *Bitters* should be incorporated in the diet – like fenugreek, bitter gourd, neem etc. which seem to help in controlling blood sugar and also bring down cholesterol.

Some common artificial sweeteners

With the availability of artificial sweeteners, diabetics can lead a sweeter existence and they can be used imaginatively to make sweets or added to beverages.

Saccharin

Saccharin is 300-500 times sweeter than sugar but leaves a bitter after taste and some experiments on rats have shown that it can lead to cancer. Although its safety has been proved in human beings, it is not very popular these days.

Aspartame

Aspartame is about 200 times as sweet as sugar. When cooked or stored at high temperatures, aspartame breaks down into its constituent amino acids and loses its sweetness. Therefore it cannot be added during cooking or to foods and beverages that are heated. It is considered safe for human consumption.

Stevia

Stevia is an herbal product that has been used for centuries in South America, and now all over the world. It is safe for human consumption.

Sucralose

Sucralose is a chlorinated sugar that is 600 times as sweet as sugar. It is produced from sucrose (sugar) and most of it passes out unabsorbed from the body. That is why it does not add to calorie intake. It is safe for human consumption.

Hypoglycemia

Diabetics should avoid fasting because their blood sugar can come down suddenly, leading to fainting or even coma. They should also learn the symptoms of *hypoglycaemia* (blood sugar coming down) and to deal with it quickly when it occurs. These symptoms may be giddiness, palpitations, sweating, headache etc. In the elderly diabetic, *these warning symptoms may be blunted*, so they should maintain regularity in checkups, meals and exercise as any irregularity can cause hypoglycaemia which may not be recognized and even lead to coma.

Exercise: Exercise is important to keep the weight under control and also to help in more efficient utilisation of sugar. Moderate exercise – aerobic and anaerobic should therefore, be actively encouraged in all diabetics.

Body Care: Diabetics need to take care of their bodies, very meticulously and examine themselves regularly, as many complications can be prevented from progressing, if detected early. They should look out for any infections, loss of sensations etc. on their skin. . Infections should be immediately attended to, as not only does diabetes increase the chances of infection, infections also increase severity of diabetes. So, don't ignore any coughs and fevers if you are a diabetic, they could turn serious.

Foot Care - a diabetic should take better care of his/her feet than his/her face! Feet should be washed daily and a lubricating cream used at night. Nails should be cut straight and not in a curved manner to prevent 'in growing'. Water at extremes of temperature (too hot or too cold) should not be poured on feet. They must never go bare-feet anywhere, and cover their feet with thick cotton socks with loose elastic and sandals or shoes. Any injuries should be immediately reported to their doctors, and they should never perform 'home surgery' on corns and boils.

Monitoring and regular check-ups - are of tremendous significance to make sure diabetic control is maintained smoothly, prevent complications and for adjustments in dosage of medications. It is also important *not to resist taking insulin if it is required to keep diabetes under control.*

Home monitoring

All diabetics should preferably have a glucometer and test their sugar at regular intervals besides testing in the laboratory once in three months.Glucometers should be standardized by taking a reading in the lab when blood is being withdrawn for testing. It must be understood that glucometer readings are taken by drawing blood from finger tips (capillary blood) which shows a higher reading as compared to the 'venous blood' that is drawn in the lab. After a few readings, it will become clear as to how much higher levels, a particular glucometer is showing and the number can be minused. In any case glucometer readings are to get an approximate idea of blood glucose levels, and regular lab testing is mandatory.

Diabetic Card - Every diabetic should carry an identification card stating roughly the following:

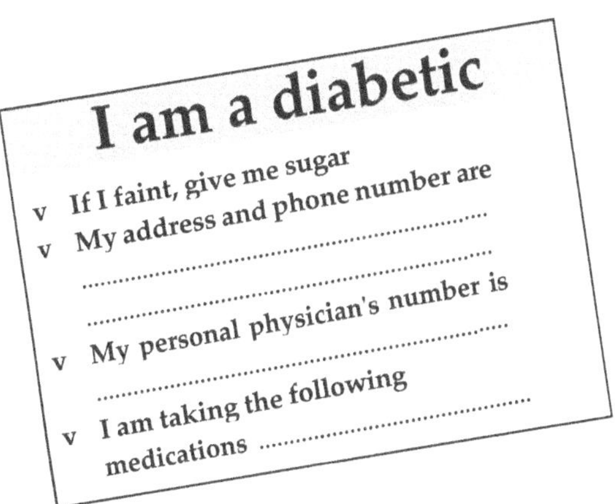

He must also carry his regular drugs and some sugar cubes with him always for use in an emergency.

Summary of guidelines for a diabetic

+ Strictly follow prescribed diet

+ Never miss a meal

+ Do not change dose of medication without consulting your doctor

+ Always carry some sweets with you in case your blood sugar goes down

+ Exercise regularly

+ Test urine & blood sugar regularly

+ Avoid alcohol & smoking

+ Avoid exposure to infections

+ Attend immediately to wounds

+ Always wear comfortable footwear & loose cotton clothing

+ Carry a diabetic card

+ Keep in touch with your physician, as newer & better drugs are constantly coming into the market

Newer methods of treatment

+ Insulin pumps are available; they are implanted under the skin and deliver insulin automatically after meals as required. They are a boon for children and the old since they avoid frequent pricks.

+ Inhaled and oral insulins are being tried.

+ Stem cell therapy in which stem cells from umbilical cords or from the patient's own bone-marrow are extracted and injected into the blood or directly into the Pancreas is another exciting new method of treatment. It is hoped that these stem cells will grow into new insulin secreting cells and cure diabetes.

+ Transplantation of Pancreas either in part or complete is also being tried.

+ Surgery for obesity that reduces size of stomach is also said to reduce severity of diabetes and even achieve a cure in some cases.

With proper care and a positive attitude, diabetics can enjoy a normal span of life. Hopefully in the near future, we will have a permanent cure for diabetes. A sweet thought indeed!

CAN DIABETES BE REVERSED?

Dibetes has always been considered incurable, irreversible, and a lifelong problem once diagnosed. Then how are we suddenly talking about its reversal? Are we talking about some new fangled treatment that has suddenly been discovered? No. Let me tell you how the thought process started, giving Diabetics a glimmer of hope-

In the last decade or so, Bariatric surgery for obesity has become very common. And in many patients after Bariatric surgery, it was found that their blood glucose came to normal, as early as within three days after surgery which had nothing to do with weight loss. In fact MRI performed within a few weeks of surgery, showed a rapid reduction in liver fat and improvement in insulin sensitivity, followed by reduction in pancreatic fat deposition and return of normal functioning of Pancreas. Fat accumulation in and around organs is how Diabetes is caused. So it got doctors thinking-

Actually it is the sudden and very drastic reduction in calories that led to these positive changes; since in bariatric surgery, you reduce the size of the stomach you can only eat so much. Now the doctors pondered, could a low calorie diet work the same way as Bariatric surgery in reversing Diabetes?

We know that insulin secreted by Pancreas, suppresses glucose output from liver. But fat inside the liver prevents this action of insulin and glucose continues to be released from liver into the blood. Excess fat from the liver spills over into the blood as fatty acids and is deposited in the Pancreas. Here it prevents insulin release after meals. Excessive fat in the Pancreas also leads to death of Beta cells that release insulin. So Diabetes is actually a disease of too much fat inside the organs and removing this fat can reverse Diabetes.

Excess of carbohydrates are also converted into fat and stored in the body if they remain unutilized for energy. Actually refined carbohydrates are a bigger culprit than fat in the diet. If we consume more fat, it can be deposited in liver, under the skin or in other organs. But consuming too much of refined carbohydrates leads to their conversion into fat that is stored only in liver.

The Counterpoint study demonstrated that a low calorie diet could reverse Diabetes. Now we can think back in reverse as to how Diabetes occurs. According to the twin cycle hypothesis, chronic and sustained high calorie diet leads to fat accumulation in liver in people who have Diabetic genes. The story begins with resistance to action of insulin in muscles. This leads to high insulin levels in blood, which in turn leads to fat deposition in liver. So a low calorie diet—(only 25% of normal calories were given for eight weeks in this study) achieved dramatic results. Not only was there a rapid fall in blood glucose, fat content of Pancreas and liver came down dramatically, with a weight reduction of about 15kg which was comparable to Bariatric surgery without the side effects of the latter.

During severe calorie reduction, the person can feel weak and giddy, but as long as he can sustain, he must continue. The diet advised should consist of 600kcals from a totally fat free diet, with complex carbohydrates and non fat proteins. Three liters of water or non fizzy, non sweetened simple fluids to assuage hunger pangs, and 200 calories from vegetables –simply cooked or in salad form. Along with diet, large muscle exercise will help in uptake of glucose by muscles, thus improving high blood sugar. Later, calorie reduction of lesser intensity, changing quality of food, and regular exercise can maintain the reversal. Once the basic cause—that is fat accumulation in liver and pancreas is removed, these organs start functioning properly again and Diabetes can be reversed.

Is it easy?

NO! But any patient with courage and a strong will power can try it under supervision of their doctor. If not complete reversal, at least a drastic reduction in medication will definitely be achieved. Continuous motivation and family support will help in achieving good results.

Precautions during attempted reversal

+ Drugs that act by secreting insulin can be stopped totally. Insulin can be gradually reduced by monitoring sugar regularly; other medicines like 'metformin' can be gradually reduced.

+ Usually a 15 kg weight loss in 8 weeks is desirable to reverse Diabetes. Those who are only slightly overweight can try to achieve a BMI that is just below normal.

+ If a patient has moderate or severe retinopathy, he should be screened after six months of beginning the attempt at reversal, since the sudden reduction in retinal blood flow associated with the return of normal blood glucose control can be bad for areas of the retina with reduced circulation resulting possibly in worsening of retinopathy

(Arun CS, Pandit R, Taylor R. Diabetologia 2004; 47:1380-84. PMID: 15309288).

For those individuals who achieve reversal of their type 2 diabetes, retinal screening should be continued for two years if there is no pre-existing retinopathy. If retinopathy is present, it should be continued until all changes come to normal.

All complications will be improved by the dietary changes. It should be noted that blood pressure and high lipid levels will also be substantially improved, with the possibility of decreasing number or dose of anti-hypertensive and lipid lowering drugs.

✦✦✦✦

14

Prevention and Management of Heart Disease

When we talk of heart disease in colloquial terms, we generally mean athero sclerotic heart disease. Now what is atherosclerosis? . "Athero' means blood vessel and 'sclerosis' means hardening. Our arterial system is like a water supply and drainage system and as long as the passage is smooth, and fluid passing through it is thin, no deposition will take place in it. Now suppose the walls of our drainage channel become rough and / or the fluid passing through it becomes thick, deposition of substances from the fluid will take place along its walls, and once this process starts, more and more deposition will continue, till there is a 'block' or choking up. This is what happens in our arteries. It may be due to damage to the vessel wall, smoking, or thickening of blood due to increased fat content, actual process being very complex, but this is to give you an idea of how it occurs. The sequence of events is probably, first the bad fats, then the cells, and finally calcium. Once calcium is deposited, the atherosclerotic 'plaque' (or patch) hardens and it may be difficult to reverse or bring it to normal without interventional methods (described below).There are many blood vessels supplying blood to the heart, and when one of these gets partially blocked, blood supply to part of the heart suffers, leading to chest pain only on physical effort, which comes to normal at rest—this is called *'angina'* If this process continues, leading to *total* block, obviously the patient will have pain at rest too---this is called myocardial infarction or as you know it - *'heart attack'*. Atherosclerosis is a normal, slow process of aging, but can be hastened by various factors. These are:

1. Obesity or over weight, especially around the tummy
2. Wrong diet
3. Dyslipidaemia
    (wrong balance of good and bad fats in blood)
4. Oxidative damage
5. Stress
6. Sedentary lifestyle
7. Smoking and alcohol
8. Blood pressure and diabetes
9. Infection
10. Some other causes -   a)   Hyperhomocysteinaemia
                          b)   Hyperinsulinaemia
                          c)   Hyperfinrinogenaemia

If we want to reduce our chances of getting a heart attack, we must correct all the factors mentioned above. So how do we go about this? Let us take it step by step.

1. **Obesity:**

    Over weight people are prone to hypertension, diabetes, & dyslipidaemia, which are all independent risk factors, and besides this, they are usually sedentary, so their blood vessels and heart have to put up with more strain. IBW (ideal body weight) can be achieved by taking small regular meals four times a day, plenty of water, salads, vegetables and sprouts (see chapter on obesity).

2. Diet

Intake of non-vegetarian food, refined sugars, refined cereal meals and saturated fats are bad for the heart. Vegetarian diet high in fibre, and whole meal cereals are good, as is fish.

Fibre: intake of soluble fibre, --- like psyllium,fenugreek, oats, barley, raisins, beans, carrots, papaya and guava; and insoluble fibre ---like skins, peels, husks, core and seeds of fruits and vegetables are very important. Fibre gives a feeling of fullness, provides bulk to stools (thereby preventing constipation) *traps e/cessive fats, and throws them out in stools,* prevents sudden rise in blood glucose, and has zero calories, so make sure you eat a fibre-rich diet.

Fruits, vegetables and legumes*:* At least 500 grams per head of fruits, vegetables and legumes including sprouts should be consumed daily. They provide vitamins, minerals, fibre and negligible calories besides anti-oxidants.

Correct balance of carbohydrates, fats and proteins-

this should be 60: 20: 20

a. **Fats** are made up of fatty acids which may be EFA (essential fatty acids) which cannot be synthesized by the body & have to be supplied from outside, & NEFA (non essential fatty acids) which are synthesized by the body. Fats can also be classified into SAFA, PUFA, or MUFA -

1. SAFA (saturated fatty acids) --- ghee (clarified butter), butter, mayonnaise, coconut oil and margarine, contain saturated fatty acids and should be avoided.

    Hydrogenation of vegetable oils leads to their

solidification thus increasing their shelf life but in the process, destroying nutrients, with addition of TFA (Trans fatty acids), which interfere with formation of EFA (essential or good fatty acids) in the body. E.g. of hydrogenated oils are- Margarine.

2. PUFA (poly unsaturated fatty acids) This may be PUFA – 6 or PUFA –3

    Pufa- 3 fatty acids are good for the heart (*also called omega –3 or essential fatty acids*) and are present in rice- bran, fish, Soya and rape seed oils and to some extent in other unsaturated oils. They are also present in green leafy vegetables, sprouts, & algae. Omega –3 fatty acids are not only good for the heart, but also required for proper functioning of the brain.

3. MUFA (Mono unsaturated fatty acids) are *good for the heart* & present in olive, canola, dark green leafy vegetables, & nuts like peanuts, almonds, cashew, etc.

    We can achieve correct balance of these oils by taking a mixture of oils, like peanut, mustard, sunflower, Soya, sesame, rice-bran and safflower oil. Or we can alternate usage of these oils.

4. **Dyslipidaemia:** - or increase in bad fats (like LDL, Triglycerides, lipo -proteins) and decrease in good fats (HDL cholesterol) should be corrected by proper diet and medication.

5. **Oxidative damage**: Oxygen, that wonderful life giving gas can actually turn toxic. During normal chemical activity in the body, certain 'free radicals' are released including *'free o/ygen'* or oxygen minus one of its electrons and *hydro/yl and supero/ide dysmutase.ions,* These free radicals turn into 'rogue molecules' and go berserk, trying to regain their lost electron, and in the

process, attack healthy cells, causing damage. 'Scavenging' these free radicals by use of 'anti-oxidants' can control and prevent this damage; examples of anti-oxidants are Vitamin C, B-carotene, Vitamin E, and Selenium etc. These vitamins and minerals therefore help in preventing heart disease and also other chronic diseases. In case of heart, they probably prevent the free radicals from combining with bad (LDL) cholesterol, leading to deposition in the blood vessels and thus 'atherosclerosis'.

6. **Stress**: Stress plays an important role in causation of heart disease, by inducing release of certain hormones, which have a deleterious effect on the heart. We have all, I am sure, heard of people suffering from a fatal heart attack on hearing some tragic news. So it is very important to combat stress with adequate sleep, yoga, meditation, exercise, and by understanding our limits and working to our capacity.

7. **Sedentary lifestyle**: Or lack of exercise, makes us obese, prone to blood pressure and diabetes besides causing lack of tone and conditioning of heart. Aerobic and anaerobic exercises are required and walking five kilometers at least five days a week is generally considered the best and safest.

8. **Smoking and alcohol**: Definitive studies are there to implicate smoking (cigarette, cigar, oral tobacco intake or even passive inhalation) as one of the proven risk factors for heart disease. Alcohol in moderation especially certain red wines are said to be beneficial for the heart, but alcohol is addicting and 'moderation' is difficult to define. Certainly, alcohol intake can lead to other problems like central obesity, which are bad for the heart. Much needs to be done to educate teenagers about the addicting effects

of smoking, alcohol intake and tobacco chewing, as they are most vulnerable to glamorous advertisements and once hooked, find it difficult to give up. This may be one of the causes of increase in heart attacks at a young age.

9. **Blood pressure and diabetes**: Uncontrolled diabetes and blood pressure are independent risk factors for heart disease. It is important for patients to keep them under control to prevent not only cardiac (heart) complications, but also those of kidneys, blood vessels and eyes.

10. **Infections:** There have been studies revealing presence of certain bacteria in the atheromatous plaques inside the blood vessels. It is assumed that these bacteria may have some role to play in the process of atherosclerosis and so eradicating them, may prevent heart disease.

11. **Some more causes**:

Homocysteine:

It is an amino acid normally present in the blood and is utilized by the body to make protein and to build and maintain tissue. Studies indicate a link between high plasma levels of homocysteine and an increased risk of stroke, certain types of heart disease, and peripheral vascular disease. Raised levels may be associated with four times higher risk than in those with normal homocysteine levels. The exact mechanism of its action isn't clear and as with CRP (see below), it's not known if homocysteine is a cause of cardiovascular disease or a marker of its presence. Recent work suggests that increased homocysteine levels may eventually cause the tissues lining arteries to thicken and scar. Cholesterol can build up in those scarred areas, providing a surface for blood clots to form. There's no consensus on what homocysteine levels are optimal, but in general, less than 12 micromoles is desirable. Readings in healthy people can range between 5 and 15 micromoles. Elevated homocysteine levels can be decreased by dietary supplementation of folate, a type of vitamin B. Foods rich in folic acid are – tomatoes, green beans, spinach, lady's finger, lentils, and black-eyed peas.

Fibrinogen:

Although fibrinogen is needed for normal blood clotting, its increase may promote excessive clumping of platelets and can result in thrombosis in an artery, leading to a heart attack or stroke. Besides inactivity, excessive alcohol consumption and estrogens, whether from birth control pills or hormone therapy, which elevate fibrinogen, smoking is the most significant lifestyle factor that raises fibrinogen levels. The normal range for blood (serum) fibrinogen is 200 to 400 mg/dL, and levels around 400 mg/dL are associated with a two-fold increase in risk of heart attack or stroke.

a) Lipoprotein :

It is formed when a low-density lipoprotein (LDL) cholesterol particle attaches to a specific protein. Studies show that an increased level of Lp(a) is associated with an increased risk of cardiovascular complications, including early coronary heart disease, heart attack and stroke. Elevated Lp(a) level, generally do not respond to most lipid lowering agents but niacin, omega-3 fatty acids or estrogen may help in some cases.

b) Hyperinsulinaemia

It is a condition where there is high level of insulin in the blood, leading to obesity, diabetes and atherosclerosis. Some medicines called *insulin sensitisers* are useful for this problem.

C-reactive protein: (CRP) is a protein produced by the liver as part of the normal immune system response to injury or infection. CRP is an inflammatory marker and inflammation has a central role in atherosclerosis leading to the accumulation of plaques of fats, cholesterol and other material in the arteries. High levels of CRP in the blood have been associated with an increased risk of cardiovascular disease, including heart attack and stroke. Low risk: Less than 1 mg/L, Average risk: 1 to 3 mg/L, High risk: Over 3 mg/L. If the CRP is greater than 10 mg/L, it's likely the result of an infection or other condition and isn't useful in assessing the cardiovascular risk and the test should be repeated in about two weeks, or after the infection is gone, to assess cardiovascular risk.

Athero sclerotic heart disease is supposed to be the commonest in South-East Asians, but with proper lifestyle modification (as outlined above), it is possible to prevent and even reverse the process and thus prevent heart disease.

So whatever the risk factors, *life style modification* should always accompany any medication for a patient of athero sclerotic heart disease.

Now there are various methods of surgically and non -surgically treating AHD. You may like to understand these newer techniques.

A) Angioplasty (also called PTCA) Here a guided wire is passed via a major artery to the blocked site, and a balloon attached to it is positioned there, and inflated. This breaks the plaques causing obstruction, and clears the block. That is why it is also called balloon angioplasty.

B) Stenting - after angioplasty, a spring like contraption called *stent* is left at the spot to maintain patency and prevent reblocking. Drug eluding stents are also available, that prevent thrombus formation inside it.

Newer radioactive impregnated stents are now available, which by emitting continuous very low levels of radiation prevent re-occlusion to a greater degree than currently available stents

C) CABG - (Coronary arterial bypass graft surgery.) Here by means of open-heart surgery, a piece of a major vein is used to bypass the blocked site hence its name. Recently, arterial grafts are being used, as venous blocks were found to reblock fast.

NOW HERE ARE A FEW PICTURES DEPICTING THE SEQUENCE OF EVENTS AFTER A HEART ATTACK

Clear Artery

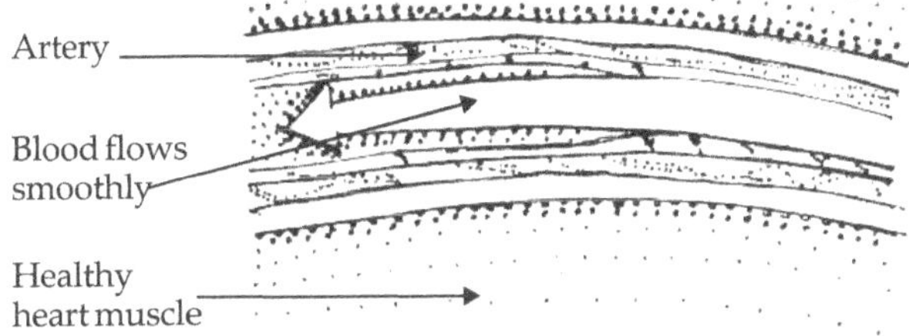

Blocked Artery

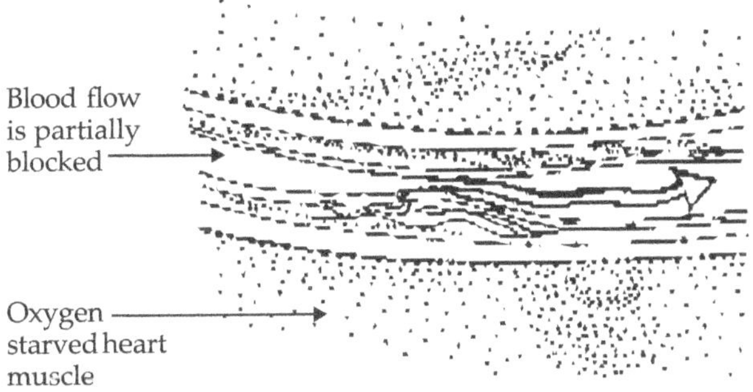

IMPORTANCE OF GOLDEN HOUR

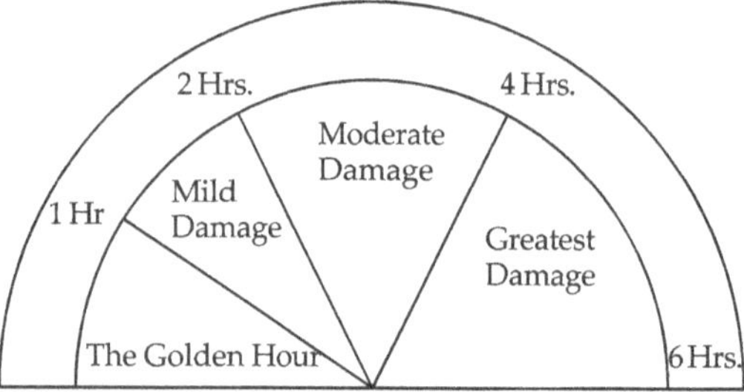

During a heart attack, the reduced blood flow leads to damage to the heart muscle. Your goal is to get to the hospital during the **"golden hour"** to keep permanent damage to a minimum.

THROMBOLYTIC MEDICATIONS

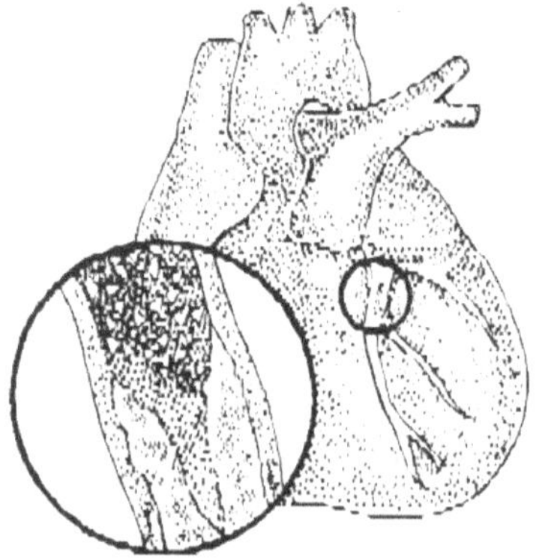

They dissolve the clots and should be used as early as possible after shifting the patient to hospital to prevent muscle damage.

ANGIOPLASTY

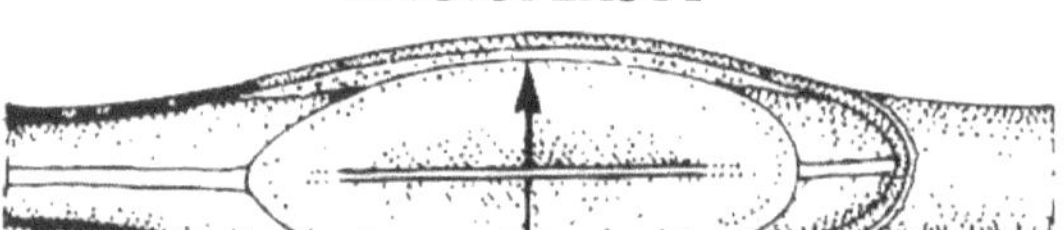

When balloon is inflated it stretches arterial wall and squashes the arterial plaques causing block.

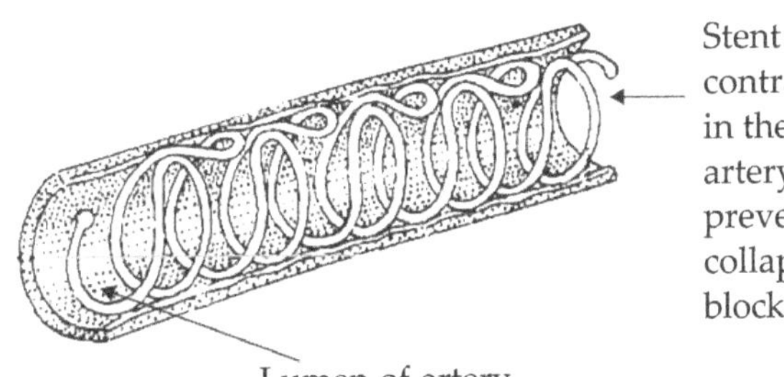

CORONARY BYPASS SURGERY

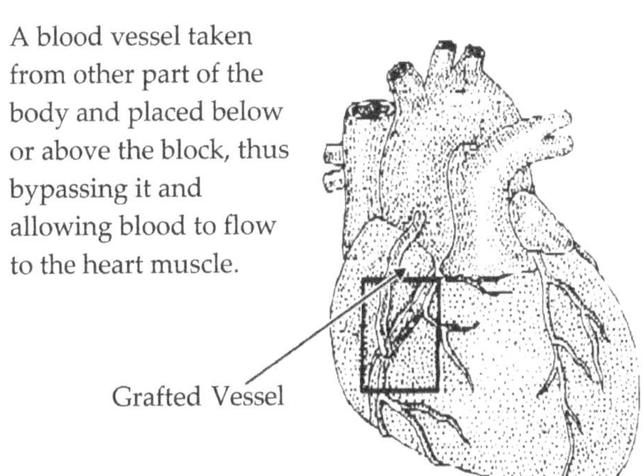

Some newer techniques: and terms

Keyhole surgery or M I C A S (Minimally invasive Cardiac surgery) For bypass grafting--also called keyhole surgery. Here incision is smaller, need for blood transfusion is minimal or not required, there is no need for heart lung machine, since it is done on beating heart, and recovery is faster special instruments being required. The beating heart is fixed by means of a contraption called octopus, so that the surgeon can operate without the heart slipping away. This is also called *Beating heart surgery.*

Batista method of myocardial revascularisation, using laser to cut channels in the heart muscles, thus supplying blood directly to them.

Arterial grafts - instead of venous grafts, arteries are being used to increase the life of the graft.

Stem cell treatment - stem cells are parent cells that can differentiate into cells of any organ. They can be derived from the umbilical cords of new born babies or from the bone marrow of the patient himself. Some studies have indicated that when stem cells are injected into the part of the heart that has blocked arteries; new vessels are able to grow and supply blood.

Choice of procedure: The big question is whether medical treatment, or intervention is required, and if so, which one. Simply because a block is detected, we need not go in for intervention.

The question to be answered is, whether the patient is incapacitated due to the block, in spite *of ma/imal medical management.*

Now the second question to be answered is whether to go in for surgical or non-surgical intervention. In a middle aged patient (50-70 years) with left main artery involvement or multiple vessel involvement, who is totally incapacitated in spite of best attempts at medical management, surgery is the only choice, subject to its being affordable. In other cases choice between surgery and medical management is made on the merits of the case.

With surgery also, 50% of the cases will get blocked again in seven – ten year's time at the same site, sometimes earlier; besides the process of blocking will continue at other sites too.

Thus when properly indicated and if one can afford them, intervention, either surgical or non-surgical, as already discussed, can save lives and there should be no hesitation in going in for them; but the old adage still holds true about *an ounce of prevention being more than worth a pound of cure.*

You can assess your chances of getting a heart attack from this scorer.

Smoking & tobacco	Non Smoker	-	0
	Less than 20/day		2
	More than 20/day		4
Weight	Desirable		0
	10% more		2
	More than 10%		4
Excess Systolic B.P.	Less than 120		0
	120 – 140		2
	More than 140		4
Hyperlipidaemia	Minor		0
	Moderate		2
	Severe		4
Physical activity	Regular Vigorous		0
	Moderate		2
	Sedentary		4
Stress & tension	Rarely tense		0
	2-3 times a day		2
	Extremely tense		4

SCORING

0 - 4	Low risk of heart attack
5 - 9	Below Average
10 - 14	Average
15 – 20	High
21 – 24	Very High

Some terms explained which you might have heard about:

Pace maker-

There is a part of the heart called S.A. NODE, which normally generates the electrical impulse, from where it is conducted to the rest of the heart. The S.A. Node thus sets the pace or beat of the heart at a particular rate and rhythm and hence is called pacemaker. Due to various reasons, some extraneous sources may start beating at a different though stronger beat and dominating the S A Node. This may be faster, slower regular or irregular. When this happens, there are some medicines which can set things right but if they fail, then an artificial pace-maker can be used which sets the pace at a programmed rate. Pacemaker can be external or implanted inside the body, and works on a battery

Electrical 'ablation'

When there is any abnormal electrical activity from an area in the heart leading to disturbance in rhythm of heart rate, it can be electrically burnt or 'ablated' so that the abnormal focus is destroyed and normal rhythm is restored.

Defibrillation- when the rhythm of the heart beat goes haywire and very irregular (especially ventricular rhythm), sudden death may occur. An external defibrillator can restore the normal rhythm and in those patients who have repeated attacks, internal defibrillator may be fitted which immediately gets activated whenever this happens, and corrects the rhythm. Incidentally most patients with heart attack die due to ventricular fibrillation and ready availability of an external defibrillator can save many lives.

Auricular-fibrillation:

+ This is irregularity in the atrial (upper chamber) rate. It can lead to formation of clot, which can dislodge, and subsequently block the brain blood vessels, leading to paralysis. It is common in patients of rheumatic heart disease. Here again, some medicines may help, failing which the cause of the irregularity has to be attended to or defibrillation can be done, or some newer procedures like M A Z E are done. Here zigzag cuts are made in order to confuse the aberrant (extra) impulses and let the regular impulse once again take over or electrically the point is ablated (burnt) and a pacemaker installed.

M V P or Mitral valve prolapse is extremely common, especially in forty plus ladies. Although it is a problem of the heart, it is not serious. Here one of the valves of the heart (mitral valve) becomes lax and prolapses into the ventricle (big chamber of the heart), thus not closing when it should and allowing blood to flow in reverse direction. This leads to attacks of palpitations - (fast beating of the heart) which the patient finds uncomfortable. In most cases, reassurance, exercise and if necessary, mild medications will help, and there is no need of any operation. Many of you will be having this problem, so I thought it is useful to explain what it means, and remove the 'cardiac phobia' attached to it.

Endo balloon surgery – using end – balloon (like in angioplasty) valvular surgery, and also closure of some congenital gaps in heart can be done, with various prosthesis (contraptions) which clamp onto the part in a spring like fashion, thus closing gaps and leaking valves. Here again, major surgery is avoided.

Transplantation of heart- a non-functioning heart can be replaced with a mechanical one (Jarvik heart), an animal one (especially from a pig,) or from a human donor. The procedure is still in the experimental stages, with no long term survivors in those who have undergone it.

✦✦✦✦

15

Thyroid Gland (Our body's thermostat)

Thyroid is a small butterfly shaped gland in the neck, just below the Adam's apple, which plays an important role in regulating metabolism (i.e. energy production and consumption) in our bodies, by secreting two hormones called T-3 and T-4.

When the levels of these hormones increase in blood, there is hyperactivity of all our body functions and conversely, if the secretions decrease, there is hypo-activity leading to reduced energy levels and a general slowing down of all our systems.

Thyroid gland is in turn controlled by the pituitary gland (in the brain), which like the conductor of an orchestra, controls all glandular secretions in the body. It stimulates the thyroid gland by means of a hormone called TSH.

If T-3 and T-4 levels (secreted by Thyroid gland) become too high in the blood, they inhibit TSH secretion from the pituitary, thereby preventing further rise in hormonal levels. Thyroid gland is the thermostat of our body, which sets the pace for all our activities, slowing down and speeding up, as required. This thermostat mechanism is controlled by thyroid –pituitary-axis, and if there is a problem at either end, we can have either hypo or hyper function of thyroid.

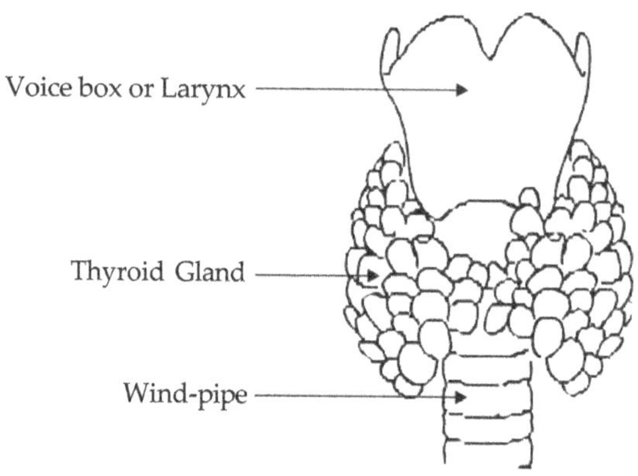

Enlargement of thyroid gland

Thyroid enlargement can be with or without change in its functions. It may increase in size due to

a. Goiter (caused by iodine deficiency)

b. Infections or reaction to infections

c. Nodules or lumps which may or may not be cancerous

   If you have a swelling in the neck, which moves with the act of swallowing, it is a thyroid swelling, and should be brought to the notice of your doctor.

Iodised salt and iodine

Iodine requirement is 100-300 micrograms a day, and if the soil in which food is grown is deficient in iodine, we can get thyroid goiter, mental retardation and even myxoedema (hypo-function of thyroid) Iodisation of salt has done away with this problem to a large extent, but consuming *large amounts* of iodised salt or sea –food can lead to both hypo and hyper thyroidism especially in the elderly, in whom it can sometimes even cause nodular enlargement which may turn cancerous.

Intake of cabbage, turnip, broccoli, cauliflower, soya, maize, tapioca and sweet potatoes increase the body's requirement of iodine.
Ref: Vegan society

Hyper function of Thyroid

When there is unbridled rise in TSH (from pituitary), or T-3 and T-4 (from thyroid), which cannot be checked by the thermostat mechanism, it results in hyperthyroidism.

Complaints- these will be due to increased metabolic activity for e.g.,

1. Diarrhoea and hyper acidity

2. Hair fall

3. Tremors or trembling of fingers and tongue

4. Increased sweating

5. Nervousness and irritability

6. Palpitations (being aware of ones heart beat)

7. Heat intolerance

8. Lack of sleep etc.

Treatment - can be with medicines (which inhibit thyroid secretions,) surgery, or radioactive iodine therapy (which causes permanent suppression of thyroid secretions, with need for life long hormone replacement).

Caution – Avoid iodized salt, and other iodine containing drugs and chemicals (like food preservatives, multivitamin pills, cough syrups, certain tonics, some dyes which are used to study kidney and gall bladder, and drugs like amiodarone, used for certain heart problems and lithium which is used for schizophrenia). Iodised salt contains Iodide in very minute doses, so the general contention of most doctors is that it can be continued in patients suffering from hyperfunction of thyroid but my personal choice is not to advocate it in these patients.

Now let us understand what happens if thyroid secretions reduce –

Hypo function of thyroid

This is extremely common especially in women. It may be due to

1. Goiter

2. Following thyroid surgery

3. Following radioactive iodine treatment for hyper function of thyroid

4. Hereditary

5. Over-intake of iodine from various sources (already discussed) or

6. After radiation to neck, for other cancers

Complaints will be due to slowing down of all functions like:-

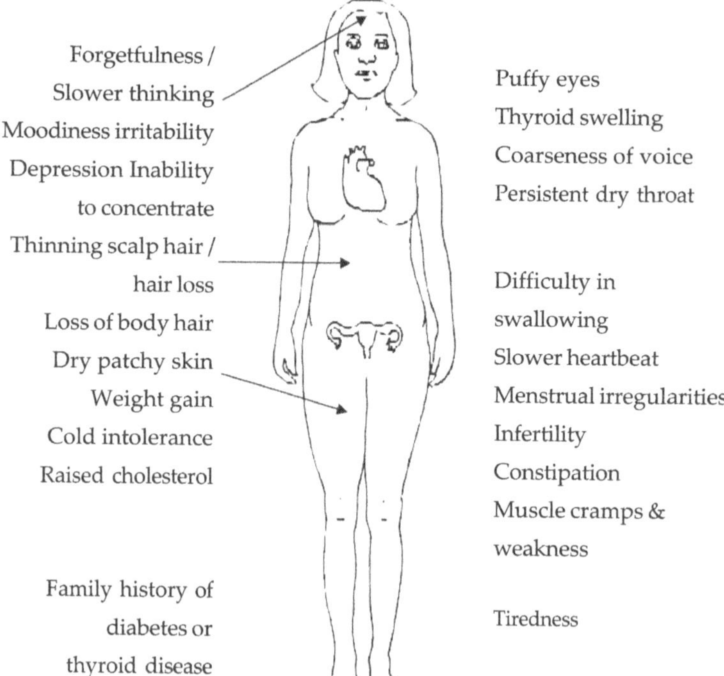

Thyroid Gland (Our body's thermostat)

Treatment is by replacement of thyroid hormone.

Diet –as for Goitre.

♦ ♦ ♦ ♦

Part – III

Problems
which may affect
only some of us

16

Allergy and Asthma

When our body is confronted with any foreign substance, a mechanism is set in motion, to counteract its ill effects, by creating a defense against it. This is called *"immunity"*. However this protective reaction can sometimes become excessive and create a disease like condition, which is called *"Allergy"*. Allergy can therefore be described as a heightened reaction of the body to external agents, which are harmless to normal or non-allergic individuals.

What are the common causes of allergies?

These may be

a.   Food items - like eggs, milk, fish and marine food, wheat etc.

b.   Animal and vegetable matter - like fur, hair, and excreta of animals or plant material.

c.   Occupational or job-related causes – working in industries like cotton, chemicals, smoke emitting industries, cement etc.

d.   External triggers- like dust, smoke, pollen, mites, fumes etc.

e.   Psychological or stress-related

f.   Exercise.

What are the tests for allergy?

Various tests can help us in detecting allergy. Some of them are: -

1. **Skin prick tests**

    Some common allergens are injected one by one into the skin and their reaction is studied. We can thus come to know about the allergies, that are likely to affect us, and hence avoid them.

2. **Immunity tests**

    As explained already, immunity is a protective reaction to foreign substances and the level of certain "immunoglobulins" in the blood can measure it. Based on these levels, we can judge the degree of allergy.

3. **Breathing tests**

    Since allergy and asthma can lead to obstruction in the breathing passages, certain tests can detect the degree of obstruction and help in diagnosis and choice of treatment.

| Predicted Average Peak Expiratory Flow Rate | | | | | | | | | | |
| Normal Males | Height in Inches | | | | | Normal Females | Height in Inches | | | | |
Age	60	65	70	75	80	Age	55	60	65	70	75
20	554	602	649	693	440	20	390	423	460	496	529
25	543	590	636	679	425	25	385	418	454	490	523
30	532	577	622	664	686	30	380	413	448	483	516
35	521	565	609	651	695	35	375	408	442	476	509
40	509	552	596	636	680	40	370	402	436	470	502
45	498	540	583	622	665	45	365	397	430	464	495
50	486	527	569	607	649	50	360	391	424	457	488
55	475	515	556	593	634	55	355	386	418	451	482
60	463	502	542	578	618	60	350	380	412	445	475
65	452	490	529	564	603	65	345	375	406	439	468
70	440	477	515	550	587	70	340	369	400	432	461

a. **P E F R - Peak Expiratory Flow Rate**

This is the commonest test. Here a cylindrical graduated instrument is used to measure the maximum amount of air, which can be breathed out after taking a full breath. If it is less than the normal range, it indicates asthma. All severe asthmatics should learn to use one and carry it with them.

b. **Spirometry and lung volume studies –**

These are more sophisticated studies providing a lot of information, which help in management of asthma.

c. **Eosinophil count in blood –**

Sometimes a routine blood test can reveal an increase in one type of cells called eosinophils, which is an indicator of allergy. At times, a high eosinophil count may be an indication of a condition called "tropical eosinophilia"for which very effective medications are available, leading to dramatic improvement in the condition of the patient.

Is allergy hereditary?

Yes, allergy has a strong genetic base. If one parent has allergy, there are 20% chances of the offspring having it too, and if both parents are allergic, the chances are doubled. So you see, in 50% of cases, there may be no manifestation of allergy but the defective genes may remain dormant and surface in the next generation but sometimes a person may be subjected to a very strong trigger agent and even *without any hereditary tendency*; he/she may get an attack of allergy.

What are the types of allergy?

Types of allergy vary according to the part of the body affected. The common ones are:

TYPE	PART OF BODY
Allergic rhinitis	(nose)
Allergic sinusitis	(sinuses)
Urticaria and dermatitis (eczema)	(skin)
Conjunctivitis	(eyes)
Asthma	(lungs) etc.

Now let us consider the individual types of allergies –

BRONCHIAL ASTHMA

Bronchial asthma is a condition, which manifests as breathlessness, wheeze (high pitched whistling sound when breathing) and cough, due to hyper-reactivity of the bronchi (air passages) in response to physical, chemical or biological stimuli (triggers). These triggers lead to spasm (tightening) of muscles in the air passages, excessive mucous secretions and oedema (swelling), which causes the problem. At least in the initial stages, bronchial asthma is reversible and as in other allergic disorders, there is a strong genetic component.

Complaints

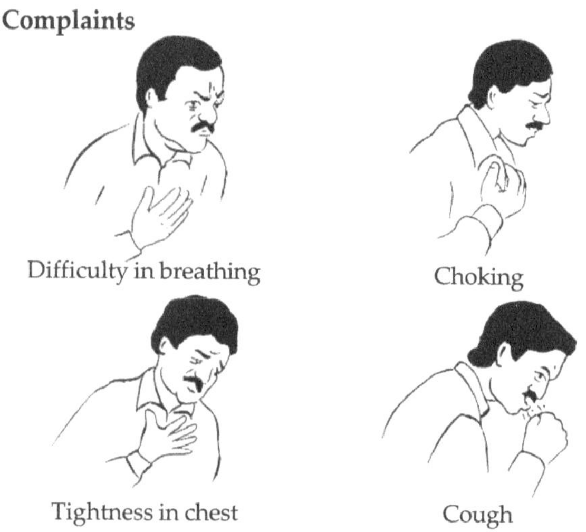

Triggers of Asthma

Besides the general triggers, which cause any allergy, there are some non-allergic causes which can set off an attack of asthma like,

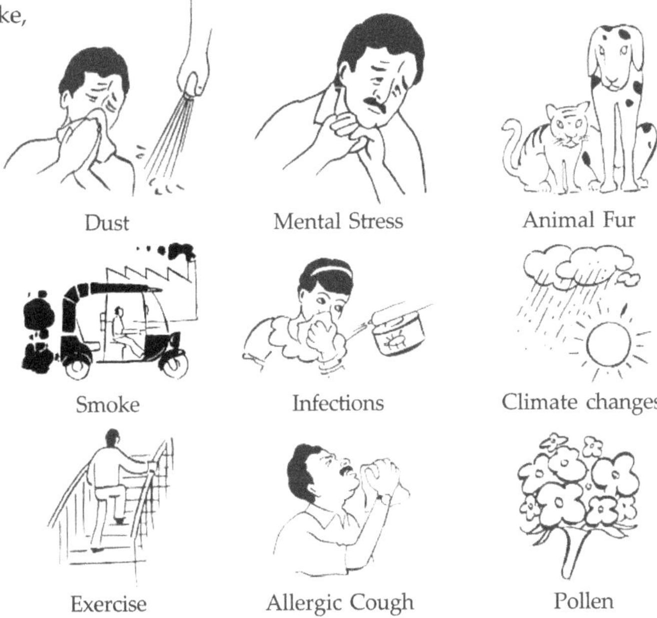

Tests for asthma

These have already been discussed -

1. Skin prick test
2. Eosinophil count
3. P E F R
4. Lung volume studies

How to reduce the frequency of the attack

- Avoid allergies
- Use mask and protective devices
- Take preventive medicines

- Protect against infections
- Avoid strenuous exercises
- Keep the head - end of bed raised with blocks
- Avoid stress

Dust mites are a common cause of asthma and it is difficult to eliminate them totally. But certain measures will help. –

1. Keep the room airy and let sunlight in
2. Avoid carpets and heavy curtains
3. Always use a clean sheet inside the rajai (comforter) or blanket
4. Don't store grains in the house and clutter the room with dust-collecting items.
5. Wear a mask when going out in dusty or polluted areas, vegetable markets etc.

Is asthma curable?

Asthma is a genetic disease, so it is not curable unless genetic modification is carried out. However in 15% of the cases, with good preventive management, a long-term attack- free status can be achieved.

Whether to use inhalers or not

Inhalers have revolutionized drug delivery in asthma, and allergy of nose and sinuses. In fact the first inhalers for asthma were probably discovered in India when "dhatura" was used as the drug and inhaled through a "hookah". In fact the hookah itself is an ingenious invention. Here the substance to be inhaled is placed in a compartment with burning coal and the resultant smoke is bubbled through water and then inhaled, thus diluting the medicine and also providing humidity (moisture), which is very useful for an asthmatic. There are many misconceptions regarding use of inhalers in asthma, so let us attempt to clear up some of them.

1. **They are expensive** - Taking a routinely prescribed tablet for asthma called salbutamol (3 tablets daily) costs us more than the same drug when taken through an inhaler. A steroid inhaler however, may be more expensive than tablets, but then tablets are 40 times more likely to cause side effects.

2. **They contain high doses of drugs** - Inhalers in fact contain 20 – 40 times *less* dose of medication as compared to oral preparations because they are targeted directly into the lungs. When medicines are given in oral form, only 1% reaches the lungs and the remaining 99% is absorbed by the rest of the body, leading to more chances of side effects like trembling and rapid pulse. Inhalers are thus safer – especially in children, pregnant ladies and the elderly.

3. **Use of inhalers indicates severe disease** - Not true again. Sometimes inhalers are given in low doses continuously to prevent severe attacks. Here again these patients are much better off than those taking tablets because they can manage with minimal dose of medicine.

4. **They are habit forming** - This is again a common misconception. Many times inhalers are given for short-term use and there are absolutely no ill effects on their withdrawal.

5. **They are difficult to use** - Once the technique is properly learnt, inhalers are easy to use and when used with *space-hulers* even children and older patients will have no problems with them.

Side effects of inhalers-

When inhalers are used for long periods without space halers, they can cause deposition of the drug in the mouth leading to local changes like ulcers and fungal infections.

Nebulisation –

here the drugs are delivered into the lungs under pressure through a mask attached to an instrument. It gives immediate relief. Home nebulisers are also available.

Travel tips for asthmatics

- Carry all medications and inhalers even if you currently do not have any problems.

- If you know how to use a peak flow meter, carry one with you, and if at any time it shows a level 35% below normal, take your medications.

- Medicines for acidity, gas and constipation should also be carried.

- Carry earplugs, protective masks (or a big handkerchief) & warm clothes.

- Use inhaler before indulging in any strenuous activity (playing, climbing, swimming etc.)

- Carry clean sheets and pillow covers to place on hotel pillow, and to use under the "rajai"(comforter) or blanket.

- Drink plenty of water.

- Carry a card declaring your asthmatic status and medications to be administered in an emergency.

- Check into hotel rooms with phone /call bell or both.

- Avoid exotic, untried foods especially seafood.

Ill effects of steroids

Steroids are hormones, normally present in our bodies and supplementing them from outside can help in allergies and asthma.

Many of you may be taking oral steroids in tablet form. You must understand that your doctor would have weighed all the pros and cons before prescribing them. Sometimes, short courses of steroids are given in severe attacks and quickly withdrawn. Here the chances of side effects are less. But in some cases, steroids have to be given for long-term use, as all other treatments do not work. Here they can have side effects like -

- Obesity
- Diabetes
- Hypertension
- Masculinisation in ladies
- Thinning of bones
- Increased chances of infections etc.

However, *when taken in inhaled form*, upto 4 – 8 puffs a day of a maximum of 250 micrograms per puff is safe even for long term use, and *fluticasone* containing inhalers are relatively safer.

When should an asthmatic seek emergency help?

There are certain circumstances under which asthmatics need emergency care. These may be –

1. When routine activities cannot be carried out
2. When breathing interferes with talking, eating or sleeping
3. When effect of inhalers lasts for less than 3 hours
4. When peak expiratory flow rate is less than 30% of predicted value

5. When there is exhaustion, confusion, perspiration or rapid pulse

6. And if you see a blue skin - **rush!**

Can an asthmatic exercise ?

As already discussed, exercise can precipitate an attack in an asthmatic, but mild to moderate exercise steadily increased, is good for all asthmatics irrespective of their severity. In fact in one Olympics, the American contingent was said to have won 23 medals (16 golds) through their asthmatic athletes. As long as proper warming up is done and inhaler is used before it, exercise cannot harm, and in fact can improve general efficiency and immunity.

Do asthmatics die young ?

No. When properly managed, asthmatics die *with* their disease and not *of* it, and there is no change in their life span if they take care of themselves well. Some prime examples of asthmatics that lived to their prime and performed to their potential are our first President---Dr. Rajendra Prasad, former Prime Minister--Smt. Indira Gandhi and iconic actor--Raj Kapoor, none of who ever appeared handicapped by their asthmatic status.

Air Passages in
Asthma   Treatments of Asthma

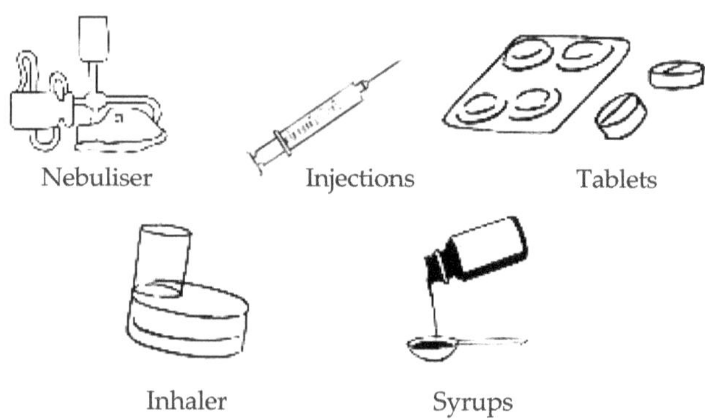

Exercises and procedures, which help in asthma

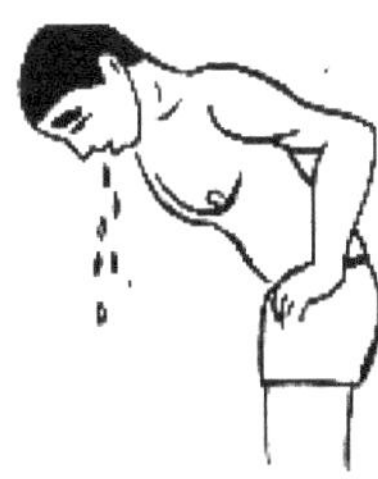

Drink 3 glasses of luke-
warm water in the
morning and vomit

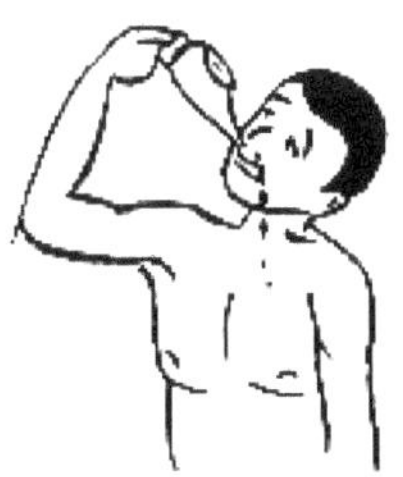

Irrigate nostrils
with warm salt
water

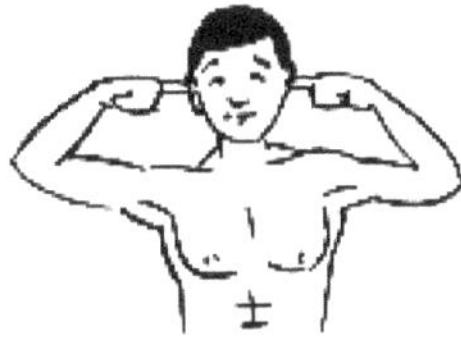

Keep both index fingers
in the two ears and recite
"omkar"OM-slowly

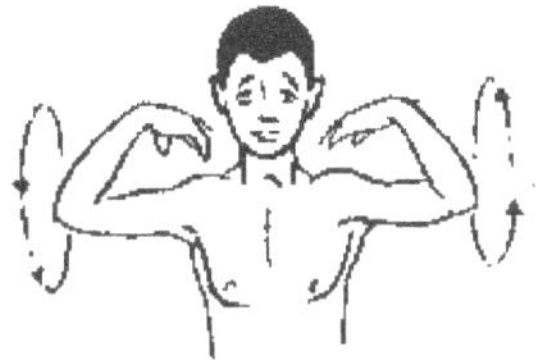

Rotate shoulders

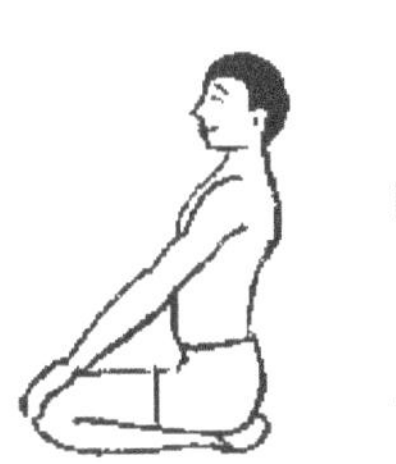

Sit on folded legs

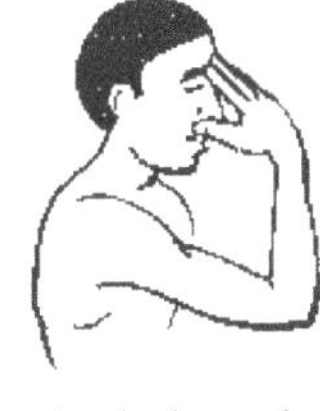

Alternatively breathe from
the two nostrils slowly,
breathing out longer than
breathing in and pausing
between the two

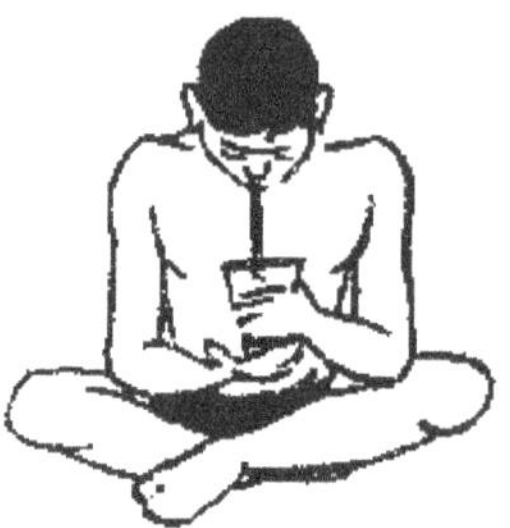

Take a glass of water
and blow bubbles in it
through a straw

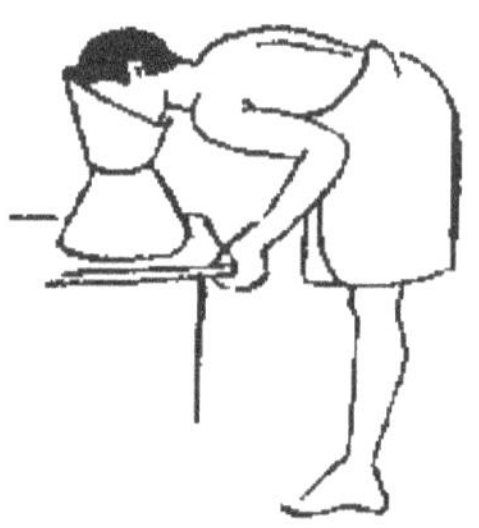

Steam inhalation

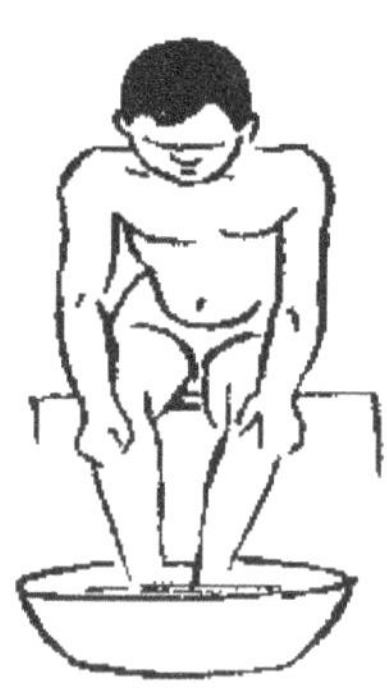

Keep the legs in warm water for 10 minutes

CHART SHOWING GUIDELINES FOR ASTHMA

+ Brush at least three times a day, cleaning the tongue, mouth and nose.

+ Gargle with salt water.

+ Don't smoke or use tobacco.

+ Avoid strenuous exercise.

✦ Avoid aspirin and anti-inflammatory drugs as far as possible.

✦ Drink plenty of water throughout the day.

✦ Avoid alcohol, cold drinks, sour fruits and unwarmed foods from fridge.

✦ Avoid carpets, pets, dust, woolen clothes.

✦ Avoid stress.

✦ Always keep medicines and inhalers at hand and be regular about medications and check-ups.

✦ Develop an exercise program to improve lung capacity.

✦ Ensure adequate sleep.

✦ Avoid heavy meals especially at bed time.

✦ Get acidity and gas treated promptly.

✦ Inform any new doctor about your asthmatic status

Ref: - Audiocassette by Dr. Virendra Singh provided by Cipla Allergy and Asthma a clinical Primer IJCP1999

✦ ✦ ✦ ✦

17

Stress and Human Body

"If you always have tears in your eyes
You will never see the light".

What is Stress?

"Stress" and "tension" have become common words, partly because of collapse of the joint family system where there was protection and support from all sides and each person did one job, and did it well. With the advent of nuclear family we feel isolated and left alone to fend for ourselves, without a higher authority to turn to in times of trouble, like a family or village head. The second cause is the "Silicon Valley Syndrome" where those who were already one up in the information stakes, have forged so much ahead economically that there is pressure on the rest of society to "keep up with the Joneses".

Can we define stress? Put simply, we can call it a "force, pressure or strain exerted upon a person who resists these forces without attempting to adapt".

Stress can be classified as domestic, social or occupational.

Domestic and social stress are inter-related, due to collapse of joint family system, exposure of those at an impressionable age to wrong influences from T.V., films and internet, increased competition for fewer "quality jobs", desire for consumer goods, increased family pressure to succeed, hassles of combined home and career management, addictions etc.

OCCUPATIONAL STRESS -

Occupational Stress is becoming very common due to interpersonal problems like sexual harassment, constant deadlines, threat of redundancy, inadequate equipment and facilities, abrasive superiors, insubordinate juniors etc.

A severely stressed person can have all three types, as stress in one place can extend over to the other two.

HUMAN RESPONSE TO STRESS

When a person undergoes stress, he may either adapt to it if he is resilient enough, or resist it. If he resists, he goes into the stage where anxiety develops and if the **stressors** persist, illness can set in.

The human body itself has a beautiful adaptation mechanism which if properly channelised can turn stress into a useful input to stimulate us into performing better.

Consider the chain of reactions set in by stress in our bodies -

Perspiration increases to keep the body cool, pupils dilate to let in more light into the eyes, respiration becomes rapid to rush in more oxygen, heart beats faster to supply more blood to the body, number of red cells increase to carry more oxygen, saliva and gastric juices dry up to enable more blood to be diverted to brain and muscles, clotting mechanism is activated in anticipation of injury, liver releases more glucose for energy, muscles tense up in preparation for action, and all the senses are heightened to prepare the body for *'Fight or flight'*.

STRESS AND DISEASE -

All stress is not bad for us. Some amount of stress is needed to keep us keyed up and make us mentally stronger, but if there is continuous or severe stress to which we cannot adapt, illness results. These are called psycho (mind) soma (body) or *psychosomatic diseases* where the body is affected by stress on the mind. There are some early warning symptoms like loss of appetite and sleep, decreased interest in surroundings and appearance, irritability, forgetfulness, new mannerisms, lack of confidence etc., which should warn us that something is wrong and take remedial action.

Psycho- somatic illnesses can be colds, migraine, hyperacidity, backache, anorexia nervosa, chronic fatigue syndrome, anxiety states, hysteria, sexual and menstrual problems, eczema (an irritant skin problem) and urticaria (hives), diarrhoea, constipation etc. Stress can also exacerbate hypertension, diabetes and heart disease. With so many preventable problems due to stress, it becomes imperative to learn how to manage it.

HOW TO HANDLE STRESS:

Attitudinal change - If we want to learn how to handle stress, the best role models should be trees. Whenever I see a tall and healthy tree standing firm on its strong foundation, swaying *with* the wind (and not *against* it), withstanding all manner of harsh conditions with resilience, while bearing bountiful fruits and flowers, I always stop to admire it. There can be no better example of how to handle stress and succeed against all odds.

Also, we must remember that when Nadia Comanenci, Sergei Bubka, Carl Lewis and Mark Spitz reached the pinnacle of their successful careers, besides talent, and dedicated practice, they had the 3 'C's of *commitment,* ability to face *challenge* and *control* over their emotions to achieve their goals, and they were also not afraid of failure. We should learn how to handle failure (since it is always *perceived* and not *real),* by learning to say "so what?" Failure should teach us what *'not to do'*, and spur us to do better in future instead of bogging us down.

Criticism is again one of the commonest causes of stress and we must learn to take it constructively by reminding ourselves that 'no one kicks a dead dog', and "a successful man is one who builds a strong foundation out of bricks thrown at him by others." Mark Twain has aptly said that there is no one successful enough, who cannot be brought down by ridicule, so we must learn how to take criticism in our stride.

In this context let me quote Abraham Lincoln whose words were framed and put up in the office of another successful world leader, Sir Winston Churchill –

"If the end brings me out right,

then what is said against me does not matter,

And if it brings me out wrong,

then ten angels swearing I am right,

Will make no difference"

Another thing to remember is - Not to worry about trivia or insignificant things since

"Small minds discuss and destroy *people*

Medium minds discuss *events* and

Great minds discuss *ideas*"

We must also know how to handle problematic situations and emerge out of them successfully. What better example to illustrate this than what the leader of the Zoroastrian Community did a long time back, when he landed on Indian shores with his band of followers at Navsari, in Gujarat. When the local king sent him a vessel full of milk indicating that there was no place for them in his state, the wise leader added sugar and sent it back, conveying the message that the Parsis would add only *quality* to the Indian nation and not *quantity*. Zoroastrians have certainly lived up to the word given by their leader, who knew how to change a situation from one where he was being rejected, to a state where he and his followers were welcomed as honoured guests.

There is a Chinese proverb which says there are thirty six ways to solve a problem out of which the easiest is to run away - successful men follow one of the other thirty five, *by facing things boldly*, since any kind of resistance can be crumbled by firm handling –

> *"Tender handed stroke a nettle*
> *And 'twill sting you for your pains*
> *Grasp it like a man of mettle*
> *And 'twill soft as soft remain"*

We should not worry either about big fish swallowing little fish or having been taken for a ride by someone, -this is how the world runs, we must just accept it and learn from our mistakes. Also don't dwell in the past or brood about the future. Channelise all your energy for the *present.* Whether cleaning the floor or developing an idea, work wholeheartedly and exclusively towards it, and remember that little drops of water end up making a mighty ocean. Don't worry about results either, diligent work should by itself be a reward; if we persevere, we are *bound to succeed.*

Dreams and desires are good for us as long as they are achievable and we learn to cut our coat according to the cloth available- so dream on, you may realise them some day.

Another important attitudinal change is to project an effective *outward image* of ourselves, since a tidy and unruffled person is more likely to instill confidence in others. A successful person is therefore one, who *like a duck, presents a calm e/terior, while paddling furiously underneath.*

One more useful dictum to remember is to –

Be Good, try to avoid harmful and negative influences (like addictions, bad company) or traits like anger, jealousy, lying etc. Remember life is like a maze- there are many paths but only one correct one, and we must learn to stick to it. Try not to develop *bad habits* and if you already have them, follow the axiom "habits cannot be thrown out of the window, they have to be coaxed down the stairs, a step at a time "(Mark Twain)

We must also learn how to interact with others, and deal sensitively with them whether they are family, servants, juniors or superiors. Each person should be treated as a different individual, like in a basket of fruits, there are some good ones and some bad, everyone has good and bad traits and we should learn to praise the good ones while tolerating the bad. Learning to *forgive* is also an art. A person who has made mistakes should be clearly told about them, the situation analysed, and then everything should be forgiven and forgotten. Also learn to bring out *others' talents* and make the best use of them. Tell people that you *depend* on them and *delegate* work wherever and to whomsoever possible.

Don't think of people as black and white - all of us have shades of grey in us--

> *'There is so much good in the worst of us,*
>
> *And so much bad in the best of us;*
>
> *That it does not behove any of us,*
>
> *To talk ill of the rest of us.*

Channelise Anger correctly and don't let it pull you down, remember temper harms us as much as it does the person it is directed at, so learn to state your case clearly and unemotionally without losing your cool. When angry we are more likely to make mistakes, which then creates more anger, becoming a vicious cycle.

Moaning and groaning is also a big 'No' for before you know it, it will become second nature to you. Nobody likes a person who is eternally complaining and it definitely creates stress in those having to live with such a person.

Develop a positive attitude and have confidence in yourself and remember the 3 'S's –

"**Start well, Step up, and Stay on it**" till you complete a job. Whenever I have a patient who breaks down totally under his emotional burden, I tell him to imagine the worst case scenario and then work UP from there. Things look better when we look upwards from the bottom of the stairs, rather than keep imagining the horrors of one day reaching the lowest rung of the ladder.

Let us emulate in real life what the highly successful software industry has come to practice; they call it *object oriented programming* technique. The salient features of this technique are as follows –

Learn to look at every situation as a new event without bringing in the past or future into the thought process. Isolate all issues into *"simple solvable objects"* and look for good people to implement them for you.

Good nutrition is also important in fighting stress and a balanced diet should consist of whole meal cereals and flours, 500 grams each of fruits and vegetables (to provide adequate vitamins, minerals and fibre), proteins from soya, fish and pulses, 5 grams. of mainly unsaturated fats, low salt, low sugar, and some spices and condiments. Reducing intake of alcohol, tobacco, tea, coffee, and avoiding smoking also help.

A successful manager of stress is therefore one who plans well, works hard to achieve his targets, balancing a his I-Q with a high EQ (emotional quotient) while keeping those around him comfortable and happy to be working with him.

Over the years, many techniques have been developed to combat stress and can be utilised by those in whom the above *attitudinal* changes do not work. Let us try to understand some of them.

STRESS MANAGEMENT II

"Acceptance is not tolerance, it is avoidance of conflict."
When a person is faced with stress, he goes through the initial shock phase, followed by a stage of resistance or adaptation and finally develops stress- related illnesses. In the first two stages, attitudinal changes alone may suffice, but in stage III something more is required and in some cases *all* available methods will need to be used to bring a person out of his problem.

These techniques can be: -

+ Improving physical fitness
+ Physical relaxation techniques
+ Mental relaxation techniques
+ Breathing techniques
+ Bio-feed back techniques
+ Seeking outside help
+ Medication

Physical fitness - Improving physical fitness (which can be achieved by walking fifteen kilometers. a week, aerobics or yogic asanas,) "tones, hones, and prevents moans and groans" – So make sure you have a sound body if you want a sound mind!

Physical relaxation – can be achieved by physical training of muscles (by experts), body massage, **and shavasana.**

Mental relaxation – Mental relaxation can be achieved by **shavasana,** meditation, listening to soothing music, reading humorous literature, chanting mantras, or saying prayers with beads or rosaries. Keeping the mind on an even keel is important to help you face choppy waters, so work towards it

Breathing Exercises - Breath is equivalent to 'Prana' or life. When someone gets a brilliant idea, he is 'inspired' and conversely when someone dies, we say he has 'expired'. From this we can gauge the importance of breath.

When breathing is efficient, it provides the body with sufficient oxygen, expels carbon dioxide and toxins, relaxes us and improves circulation. On the other hand look at the examples of inefficient breathing -

An anxious person	- breathes rapidly
A depressed person	- has "sighing" breathing
A hysterical person	- hyperventilates
And a child with temper tantrum	– holds its breath

Breathing can be abdominal, chest or clavicular types.

Abdominal breathing is the most efficient. Here the abdomen goes out when we inspire and in, when we expire. Chest and supra clavicular (collar bone) muscles are used as accessories.

In chest breathing - predominantly chest muscles are used

And clavicular breathing - comes into play when we are short of breath and need to use all muscles associated with breathing.

Some simple breathing exercises are as follows: -

1. Lie on your back with one hand on chest and one on abdomen. Practice abdomen going up in inspiration and down in expiration 12 – 16 times a minute

2. Lie on stomach with head resting on folded hands and do the same - abdomen touching the ground on inspiration and caving inwards on expiration.

3. Nostril breathing – close one nostril; breathe in and out of the open nostril 3 times. Then close the open nostril and do the same with the other one. Lastly breathe 3 times with both nostrils open. Repeat the cycle.

Bio–feed-back - Here relaxation techniques are practiced, and various parameters like sweating, pulse, blood pressure, respiratory rate, electrical activity in brain, muscle tension etc. are displayed on a screen and the patient encouraged to progressively improve his performance, based on the feed back received.

Seeking outside help –

1. Joining a social group, laughter club, towel club (each person talks about his sorrows, and everyone sympathises), listening to discourses on Bhagvad Gita, Ramayana, Bible or Koran, joining a trekking group etc. will help in reduction of stress.

2. Psychotherapy - by a trained psychologist, can benefit many people.

There is a lot of difference between a psychotherapist and a psychiatrist. A psychotherapist tries to cure the mind by various methods, especially by *influencing* a person into believing in himself and by trying to iron out all the rough edges. Management gurus also have various techniques to achieve this.

Medications – Should be only as a last resort, and by a psychiatrist. A psychiatrist is a doctor, who treats the mind with medicines and tries to restore its balance. When everything else has failed, help of a psychiatrist should be sought; and there should be no inhibitions or shame about this.

My psychiatrist colleague says he envies me, as patients do not have any inhibitions about consulting a physician for diabetes or blood pressure. Psychiatric problems are also due to chemical imbalance, just like other diseases and there is no need to look down on these patients. Many of them are now a part of mainstream society, carrying on their duties almost like normal individuals as long as they take their medications regularly and remain under medical supervision. Patients must be told repeatedly that they are no different from patients of blood pressure or diabetes who also have to take life-long medication to be able to carry on their daily activities. Once the family and the patient are properly counseled into *accepting* the problem, management is easier. Later on, as improvement occurs, other techniques should be added to help in maintaining cure, but preferably under psychiatric supervision.

Now there are certain conditions, which are important, because apparently they seem to be physical problems but actually have a psychological background. A few of them are -

A) Munchauson's syndrome:

Count Munchauson was born in Europe long ago, and although

not so famous as another European Count - (Dracula), he is equally important, because a disease has been named after him. Munchauson although extremely healthy, went from one apothecary (doctor) to another, with imaginary and changing complaints each time. If one doctor lost interest in him, he quickly switched over to another. Patients of Munchauson syndrome change their complaints, so that repeated consultations and investigations are a never-ending requirement. They can be extremely cunning too, so that it is difficult to judge whether their problems are real or not. I had a patient who used to vomit two to three times a day, on whom we tried every possible medical management. – Eventually even admitting her to hospital and investigating her thoroughly. Every kind of specialist was called in, but we drew a blank – the vomiting continued and my standing with the relatives of the patient continued to plummet. Luckily (for all of us) a nurse one day caught the patient self-inducing her vomiting, and a psychiatrist was called in. Her dramatic improvement with his medication was really remarkable

A) CFS: CFS or chronic fatigue syndrome is another condition with a psychiatric background. Here, the main complaint is weakness. After huge amounts of money & time are spent and numerous investigations done, we reach this diagnosis. These patients are hard to cure, and need intensive psychotherapy and continuous motivation, to make them come out of their morbid fatigue. A lot of patience is needed, both on the doctor's part, and also on the part of the family to achieve positive results.

A N: Anorexia Nervosa is usually seen in younger people, but with increasing trends towards looking good and maintaining perfect figures, especially with actors becoming role models, more and more people will be presenting with this condition even in their middle age. Here the patient will go to any lengths

to remain thin, including starving and inducing vomiting –
sometimes even courting death in the process (as happened to
one of the singers from the group 'carpenters')

Bulimia

It is the reverse of Anorexia nervosa. Here the patient goes into
binges of eating, in ancient Roman style, and even progressively
increasing tyres around his / her waist, do not stop these orgies.
A lot of effort is needed to bring these patients out of this
problem.

So if you have any of these cases at home (Munchauson, CFS, AN
or Bulimia), recognise the fact that they may require psychiatric
help.

CASE – STUDIES

1. Ms. X was a normal girl doing well, when over a period of
    time she started showing symptoms (complaints) of
    aggression, withdrawal from society, suspicion of near
    and dear ones etc. all pointing to a mental problem called
    Schizophrenia. Luckily for her, her mother (who bore the
    brunt of her violence) understood the problem and
    approached the family doctor, who then referred her to a
    psychiatrist and medication was given to the patient
    surreptiously disguised in food. When the patient's
    condition improved, she was willing to visit the
    psychiatrist on her own, and was slowly rehabilitated.
    Although not 100% like other people (she still gets
    periods of mild withdrawal) she is able to be an active
    member of the society and carry on with her profession,
    at a moderate level with continuous motivation and
    encouragement from her family along with regular
    check-ups with her psychiatrist.

2. Ms. Y a brilliant and beautiful girl with a similar history

however did not fare so well, as she did not have a strong and determined parent to face her aggression with patience. There was all round neglect and avoidance of the problem by the family. With a lot of help from relatives, she has been partially rehabilitated but even now there is no effort to confront the problem, and accept it. The tragic farce continues with no regular check-ups, or intake of medication, pretence of carrying on with a job, and running away from unpleasant situations, with frequent relapses.

Illustrated above are two cases with similar problems both almost the same age. One was handled well because of the active cooperation of the family and the other case was totally mishandled. It is therefore very important for the family to recognise the problem early and seek psychiatric help. There may not be 100% improvement, but even 70 – 80% progress is noteworthy. At every step there should be no effort to push a patient beyond his/her capacity. The temptation is to think - 'O.K. now she is normal, she should take on more responsibilities.' The danger here can be a relapse. It is much better to take it slowly; step-by-step and let them function within their capability and appreciate the fact that they are soldiering on *in spite of* heavy medication and social pressures.

Ref: -

Jaggi O.P. Mental tension and its cure- Longman 1999

Pestonji D.M.-Stress and coping, the Indian experience

Patel Chandra-complete guide to stress management- MacDonald and Co. 1989

✦ ✦ ✦ ✦

18

Paralysis, Parkinson's, Alzheimer's and Epilepsy

*"Now is not the time to think of **what you do not have**, Think of what you can do with **what there is"** Ernest Hemingway*

PARALYSIS OR STROKE

If there is one fear everyone begins to have as they grow older, it is the fear of paralysis, and becoming 'dependant' on others. Stroke, is a psycho-socio-economic problem, where the mind gets depressed, the body incapacitated, social life suffers, besides the obvious economic implications. Post-stroke hospitalisation is also prolonged and expensive and even after coming home, the patient has to spend money for physiotherapy and possibly, nursing care. Family members too have to devote extra time to the affected patient for a long time, and the ultimate cost of care can be prohibitive.

Prevention therefore is very important - by controlling diabetes, blood pressure, hyper lipidaemia (increase in bad fats in blood), and cessation of smoking, regular exercise, and reduction in mental stress. Adequate mediclaim insurance should be planned in advance to avoid a sudden financial burden.

Now what are the causes of paralysis?

Paralysis can be in one limb, lower limbs, full body, one side of the body, only part of the body etc.

The causes may be –

1. Infections in brain or spinal cord.
2. Inflammation in brain or spinal cord.
3. Rupture of blood vessels.
4. Block in blood vessels.
5. Tumours or growths.
6. Trauma or injury to brain or spinal cord.
7. Due to degenerative or aging changes.

Risk factors are -

+ Blood pressure.
+ Irregularities in heart rhythm(auricular fibrillation).
+ Increase in bad lipids.
+ Diabetes.
+ Use of blood thinning and anti-clotting drugs.
+ Surgery.
+ Sudden loss of blood or fluids.
+ Smoking.
+ Old age.
+ Severe anaemia.
+ Oral contraceptives, pregnancy, childbirth, and hormonal treatment of menopause.
+ Increase in 'homocysteine'- a chemical that increases blood stickiness.
+ Anaemias due to altered shape of red blood cells.
+ Cold remedies containing PPA - phenylpropanolamine (they have been banned now).

Presentation of Stroke

+ Resulting paralysis can be in one limb, lower limbs, full body, one side of the body, or only part of the body.

+ There can also be inability to understand the spoken word or to speak, or other speech defects.

+ loss of vision to one side, loss of or abnormality in smell and taste.

+ Imbalance .

+ Altered breathing and heart rate .

+ Memory problems.

+ Lack of coordination and giddiness.

+ Headache and vomiting—more with haemorrhagic stroke.

+ The patient can also present with fits or unconsciousness.

'Silent' Stroke

A silent stroke is detected when an MRI or CT scan is performed for other things. The person may not have any complaints but there is evidence of brain damage. These patients are at high risk of a full blown stroke and should be put on intensive preventive treatment and follow up. The risk of silent stroke increases with age but may also affect younger adults and children, especially those with acute anaemia.

TIA

TIA or transient ischaemic attack is a condition where the patient suffers a temporary block of a vessel leading to minor paralytic symptoms that quickly recover. These patients are also at high risk for a full blown stroke later.

Treatment

As soon as a patient of stroke is admitted, a CT scan or MRI should be performed to differentiate between ischaemic stroke (due to a block by a thrombus) and a haemorrhagic stroke (due to bleeding).

Ishaemic stroke may occur because of thrombus developing in a blood vessel of the brain, or due to *'embolism'* i.e. a thrombus develops elsewhere, gets dislodged and is carried by the blood stream to a brain vessel which it blocks. Commonest source of a thrombotic embolism is from the heart. Besides a thrombus, embolism can also be due to other particles like fat(from bone marrow of a broken bone), cancer cells, air, or bacterial clumps.Ischaemic stroke can also be due to less blood supply, and due to severe loss of blood or fluids due to any cause.

If it is an ischaemic stroke, clot busting drugs are immediately injected and other complications dealt with. *tPA* (tissue plasminogen activator) is used to dissolve the clot and open up the artery. It should be given within three hours of the stroke in patients whose blood pressure is normal and they have not undergone recent surgery. But a few patients have been known to develop brain haemorrhage after the injection. Another injection that is being tried and is looking promising is *'alteplase'*

'Intra arterial fibrinolysis' can also be performed where these injections can be given directly into the clot site by passing a catheter through an artery into the affected brain vessel and injecting the drug.

Thrombectomy can also be performed—this is like angioplasty done for heart vessels. This is accomplished by inserting a catheter into the femoral artery in the groin, directing it into the cerebral (brain) circulation, and deploying a corkscrew-like device to ensnare the clot, which is then withdrawn from the body.

A stent (a spring like device that prevents re-narrowing of the artery) can then be placed (see the chapter on heart and cardiovascular system).

Primary prevention of an Attack

Prevention of first attack may involve the administration of antiplatelet drugs (reduce blood stickiness) such as aspirin and dipyridamole, control hypertension and diabetes, stop smoking, exercise regularly, and reduce mental stress.

Use of statins (to reduce the level of bad lipids) will also help. Selected patients may benefit from carotid endarterectomy (removing the clot) and the use of anticoagulants (blood thinners).

Prevention of recurrence of Ischaemic Stroke

Anticoagulation drugs like *warfarin* reduce recurrence by 60% but a blood test called prothrombin time has to be performed regularly. *Dabigatran* is a new drug that does not require this kind of monitoring.

Hemorrhagic (bleeding) Stroke

It generally occurs in small arteries or arterioles and is commonly due to hypertension, malformed blood vessels, bleeding disorders, and in drug addicts using cocaine and amphetamine.

Treatment of Hemorrhagic Stroke

Patients have to be monitored for changes in the level of consciousness, and their blood pressure, blood sugar, and oxygen saturation levels have to be maintained.

Stem Cell Treatment

As for other chronic problems, stem cell treatment is also being tried for stroke. Stem cells are unique and have the potential to develop into many different cell types in the body including brain cells. They also have the ability to produce more stem cells. After the stem cell therapy, positive results were achieved after an average of about 2 months from the treatment. After local injection of stem cells-(see details of procedure in next chapter on Parkinsonism), majority of the patients experienced better coordination and improved motor skills in their hands and fingers. Post treatment, patients had the ability to stand and walk without being dependant.

Stroke Rehabilitation

Stroke rehabilitation can last anywhere from a few days to over a year. Most return of function is seen in the first few months, and then improvement tapers off. However, patients have been known to continue to improve for years, regaining and strengthening abilities like writing, walking, running, and talking. Daily rehabilitation exercises should continue to be part of the stroke patient's routine. Complete recovery is unusual but not impossible and most patients will improve to some extent. Proper diet and exercise are known to help the brain to recover.

A rehabilitation team is usually multidisciplinary as it involves staff with different skills working together to help the patient. These include nursing staff, physiotherapists, occupational therapists, speech and language therapists, and usually psychologists and social workers, also.

Good nursing care is fundamental in maintaining skin care, feeding, hydration, positioning, and monitoring vital signs such as temperature, pulse, and blood pressure.

A wheelchair, walkers, canes, and other aids may be beneficial. Occupational therapist is involved in training to help relearn everyday activities such as eating, drinking, dressing, bathing, cooking, reading, writing, and toilet use.

 Speech and language therapy is appropriate for patients with the speech production disorders.

Home rehabilitation of a case of Stroke

Once the patient comes home, there are certain guidelines that can be followed to achieve a good outcome and early mobilisation. Intensive management has to continue and the physiotherapist's services should be utilised on a long-term basis as an expert, to avoid complications.

Since paralysis is mostly one-sided, the tendency is to exercise the affected side only in order to strengthen the muscles. This is wrong, as a bilateral or symmetrical approach will ensure that the patient maintains his/her sense of balance and co-ordinated movements of the body. For similar reasons, sticks and tripods should be discouraged except for a short time, if at all. Patient should be encouraged at an early stage to move away from the bedroom and dress up well to overcome the feeling of being an invalid and certain stimulation techniques can be practiced to bring about 'feeling' in the affected parts.

Stimulation Techniques
(please consult your Doctor first)

1. Ice stimulation - Placing the affected limbs in melting ice for a few seconds, reduces spasticity (tightness in muscles), and often improves movements.

2. Stroking the limbs with ice or a brush also helps.

3. Pressure tapping - tapping over the top or side of foot or hand works similarly.

4. Heel banging - With one hand on patient's knee, the heel is banged on the ground, as the patient sits on a chair.

5. Pressing a rubber ball kept in the hand to strengthen it.

6. Wringing a dry towel.

7. Electrical stimulation and vibration therapy to the

antagonist (opposite) muscles has also been used with some success.

Regular visits by a physiotherapist should continue for months to avoid wrong movements, contractures (tight muscles), swollen limbs and other complications.

Complications

Disability affects 75% of stroke survivors and most will not be able to get back into full time employment. Stroke can affect patients physically, emotionally and mentally,

Some of the physical problems that can result from stroke include muscle weakness, numbness, pressure sores, pneumonia, urinary incontinence, speech defects, difficulties in carrying out daily activities, appetite loss, speech loss, vision loss, and pain. Some patients will develop fits that can last life-long. If the stroke is severe enough, or in a certain location such as parts of the brainstem--- coma or death can result.

Emotional problems resulting from stroke can be due to direct damage to emotional centers in the brain or from frustration and difficulty in adapting to limitations in lifestyles. They include anxiety, panic attacks, apathy, lethargy, irritability, sleep disturbances, lowered self esteem, memory problems, and withdrawal from society.

Mental problems can range from depression to psychosis.

CASE STUDY

A middle-aged male with post infective paralysis of lower limbs was totally bed-ridden for six months in spite of best management. He did not lose heart and was always sure he would walk although all of us had given up hope, and after discharge he summoned up all his will power and slowly painfully he did walk and came to meet us after three months leaning on a stick!

Use of ball—**a rubber ball comes in very useful when the hands are paralysed. It should always be kept in the affected hand and an effort made to press it as often as possible.**

Physiotherapeutic Exercises (for paralysis) which can be done on one's own-
Always use support of good limb to facilitate exercises & help of attendant on stairs.

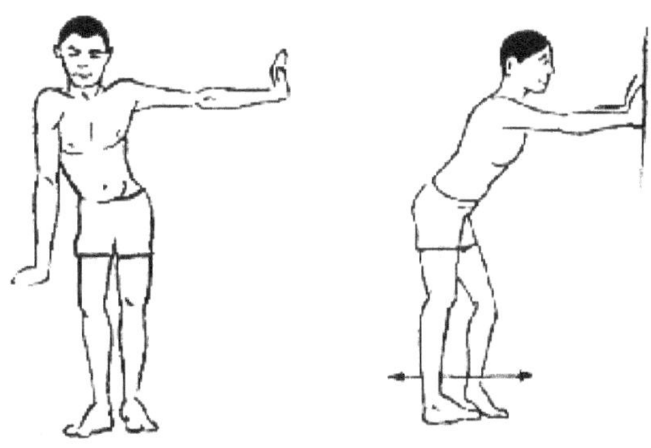

Trying to turn the body & press the wall with the hands

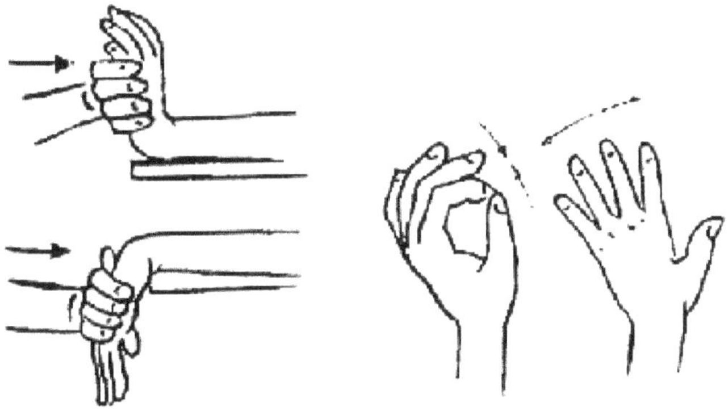

Press hand up & down against resistance provided by healthy hand

"Counting fingers" exercise

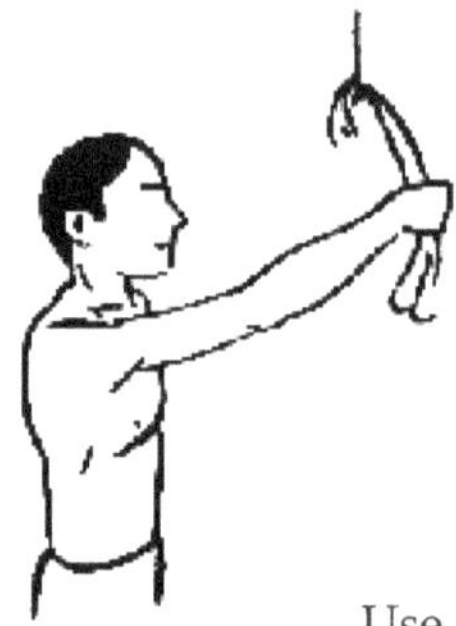

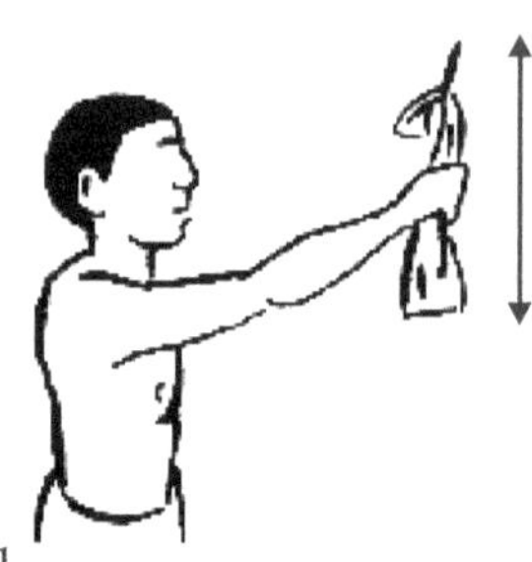

Use a towel

1) to squeeze
(like wringing out water.)

2) To "climb up"
the towel with the hands

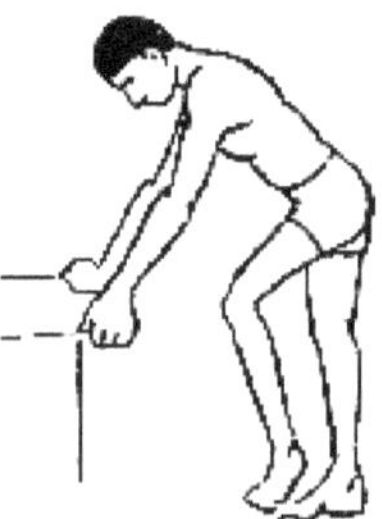

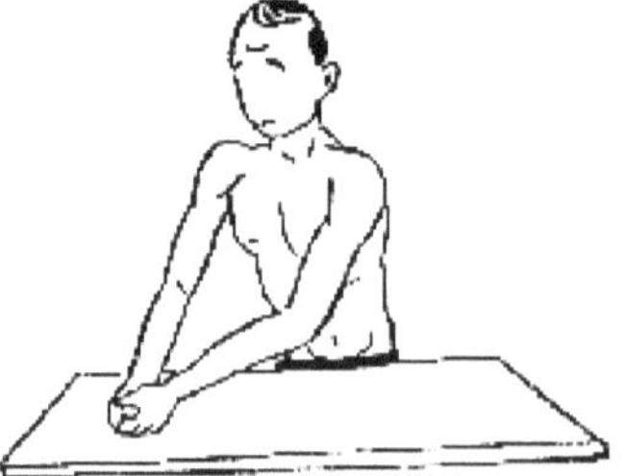

Trying to turn the
body & press the
table with the hands

Press affected hand
with good one & try
to move it against
this pressure

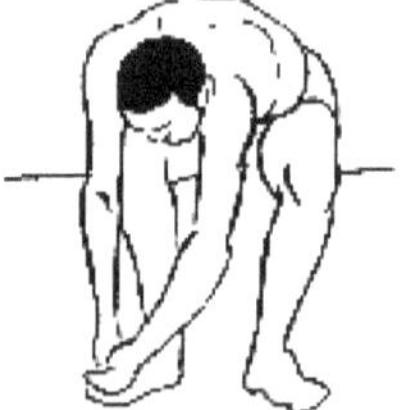

Moving clasped hands from side to side& bending
down, sitting on a chair

Katherine Bevis tells this story   There was a boy in a school who walked on crutches due to infantile paralysis, but always remained cheerful. When friends praised him for this, he said—'the paralysis has not affected my mind and heart!'

Two other common diseases of nervous system in old age are:

PARKINSON'S DISEASE

Parkinson's is a disease where there's a reduction in a chemical called *dopamine* in the brain, either due to certain infections or as a part of aging process, and rarely also due to certain drugs. This common disease was first described by James Parkinson in 1817. The disease occurs in about 1% of people over the age of 65 and the peak onset is in the sixth decade of life. There are no proven genetic factors contributing to the disease. The primary derangement in Parkinson' disease is a loss of dopaminergic neurons in the section of the brain called *substantia nigra* a part of *basal ganglia.*

The cardinal manifestations of the disease are *bradykinesia* (abnormal slowness of movement), *akinesia* (absence of movement), *rigidity or stiffness,* (often described as lead pipe or cogwheel rigidity), and *tremor* (fine movements of the hands typically seen at rest, described as "pill rolling"). In addition, a number of other findings are associated with Parkinson's including *masked facies* (blank expression), *festinating gait* (patients walk with many small steps and have difficulty starting, stopping and turning), and *micrographia* (very small writing). Mental depression may follow due to the physical problems.

It is a progressive disease where various drugs are given to replace the deficient chemical, and also to treat the symptoms. The most famous patient of this disease is of course, Mohammad Ali, the boxing champion. Medication should be kept to a minimum, just enough to keep the patient comfortable, and able to carry on with his routine activities.

After 5-10 years of treatment with drug therapy patients, often become less tolerant to the drug. They begin to experience episodes of "OFF" periods, where they have severe rigidity, akinesia, and tremor, followed by "ON" periods, when they suffer from severe dyskinesias (involuntary movements of the limbs). For many patients medical treatment becomes increasingly difficult and it is nearly impossible to find a drug regimen that adequately controls the disease without side effects. Some of these patients are then candidates for surgical therapy.

Surgery

This involves *Stereotactic* stimulation of the affected part with electrodes which is a minimally invasive surgery. Let me explain this in simple terms   A magnetic resonance (MRI) compatible *stereotactic* frame is affixed to the skull. Following frame placement, the patient is taken to the MRI scanner where multiple images are obtained first. Once the target point has been calculated, the patient is brought to the operating room, a burr hole (a tiny hole) is made in the skull and the electrode guide tube is lowered into it and guided to the affected part. High frequency stimulation of the part usually causes an improvement in rigidity and bradykinesia which may be readily appreciated during the surgery itself by using tasks such as finger tapping, rapid pronation/supination(up and down movement) of the forearm, and toe tapping. Potential problems in speech are also assessed during high frequency stimulation by asking the patient to repeat several complex phrases and noting any difficulties. Either deep brain stimulators are then implanted in the affected parts, or a small incision is made in the *'globus pallidus'* (pallidotomy) or part of the *thalamus* (thalamodotomy). After surgery or stimulation, the patient is evaluated and medication continued only as required.

Stem Cell treatment

Intense research is underway to cure Parkinson's disease especially stem cell research (stem cells are basic cells that can be grown into any part of the body.) Here stem cells from the patient's own bone marrow or umbilical cord of a newborn baby are implanted into the *basal ganglia* (the part of the brain affected in Parkinsonism), with the hope that they will multiply and form new cells that can secrete dopamine the chemical that is deficient in Parkinson's and thus cure the disease. The procedure is same as in surgical treatment. Some centers have used stem cells from the retina of eyes—*human retinal pigment cells.* A single injection of stem cells will be injected in the affected part of the brain. The treatment includes the implantation of cells into the region in the brain where the damaged cells are, along with a daily cocktail of medications that 'fertilize' this area, helping the cells to survive and keep on renewing themselves.

Stem Cell procedure

This program usually takes five to seven weeks of stay in the Hospital.

After thorough evaluation, medications are given to clear the blood vessels in the brain so that the injected stem cells will proliferate better.

Then medicines are given to 'wake up' sleeping stem cells. These stem cells (from umbilical cord, bone marrow or retina) are then harvested and injected through stereotactic surgery (already described above). After the first cycle of treatment is completed, the patient is sent home and can come back after a few months for a second cycle of treatment if required.

Non-surgical Stem Cell treatment

Stem cells, delivered intranasally (through the nose), have been found to substantially improve motor function in Parkinson's disease in a study conducted by the US Alzheimer's Research Center and the University Hospital of Tubingen in Germany. Stem cells are derived from the Bone marrow and delivered intra nasally.

Intranasal administration (into the nose) of stem cells to the brain is a promising and non-surgical alternative to current surgical procedures. It also opens up the possibility of chronic stem cell treatment (repeated), which would increase the number of cells delivered to the brain and likely enhance the beneficial effects.

Complete treatment of Parkinson's

The complete treatment includes medications, stem cell implantation procedure, surgery, biofeedback treatment (counseling) and comprehensive rehabilitation.

Next let me also tell you about another common disease of ageing called -

ALZHEIMER'S - DISEASE

It is another disease of aging, (its most well known victim being former US president Ronald Reagan who passed away recently) and was first described by German psychiatrist and neuropathologist Alois Alzheimer in 1906 and was named after him.

It is due to general depletion of nerve cells in the brain due to formation of plaques *and* tangles in the brain. It is seen in people usually after the age of 65 years although there is an early onset type seen in younger people. Alzheimer's is predicted to affect 1 in 85 people globally by 2050.

The patient complains of forgetfulness and reduction in mental faculties, which gets progressively worse. Initially the complaints are wrongly attributed to stress or old age. There is inability to acquire new memories, observed as difficulty in recalling recently observed events and the diagnosis is usually confirmed with behavioral assessment and cognitive tests(tests that evaluate understanding ability), followed by a brain scan. As the disease advances, symptoms include confusion, irritability and aggression, mood swings, language breakdown, long-term memory loss, and the general withdrawal of the sufferer from day-to day life. Other symptoms of Alzheimer's disease include agitation, depression, hallucinations, anxiety, and sleep disorders.Gradually bodily functions are lost, ultimately leading to death. The mean life expectancy following diagnosis is approximately seven years. Fewer than three percent of individuals live more than fourteen years after diagnosis.

Some drugs are being tried and are proving to be of partial benefit, like lecithin, eptastigmine, tacrine, lazaroids, piracetam, antioxidants, chloroquine, aspirin, anti-inflammatory drugs, calcium channel blocking drugs, etc. Sedatives, anti depressants and anxiety reducing medicines are also used. Aluminum has also been implicated, as a cause recently, whether rightly or wrongly we don't know - so avoid using aluminum cooking utensils just to be on the safe side.

Non-medication based treatments include maximizing patients' opportunities for social interaction and participating in activities that they can still enjoy. Cognitive rehabilitation, (whereby a patient practices on a computer program for training memory), is also being tried. Mental stimulation, exercise, and a balanced diet are suggested, as both a possible prevention and a sensible way of managing the disease. Difficulty in sleeping (insomnia) occurs in many patients with Alzheimer's disease at some point in the course of their disease. Sleep improvement measures, such as a peaceful noise free room, adequate treatment of pain, and limiting nighttime fluids to prevent the need for urination, can help.

Because AD cannot be cured and is degenerative, proper

management of patients is essential. The role of the main caregiver is often taken by the spouse or a close relative. Alzheimer's disease is known for placing a great burden on caregivers; the pressures on whom can be wide-ranging. It affects them socially, psychologically, physically, mentally and economically.

There is a lot of research going on to find a cure for Alzheimer's so hopefully in the next decade something fruitful will emerge.

Next we will talk about another common problem called — Epilepsy.

EPILEPSY

What is Epilepsy?

There are electrical waves in the brain that are normally present. And sometimes the brain generates different waves from the usual ones and these *abnormal* electrical waves stimulate the muscles in the body in an erratic fashion, inducing involuntary contractions, which we call epilepsy. The classical presentation is a sudden onset of contractions of the body with frothing at the mouth, followed by unconsciousness.

A lot of stigma is attached to a patient of epilepsy, which is totally unnecessary. It is a disease like any other and there is no need to be ashamed of it. The first time a patient has an epileptic attack, he should be fully investigated to find out if there is a treatable cause.

The causes may be -

+ A tumour or space-occupying lesion, which is triggering the attacks.

+ Certain infections

+ Worm infestations that form a 'cyst' in the brain.

+ A mal-formation in a blood vessel that ruptures

+ Sometimes it can occur due to the scar formation after an infective focus heals

+ Due to low blood glucose

+ High fevers,

+ High blood pressure—leading to rupture of a blood vessel

+ Low blood calcium,

+ Electrolyte imbalance,

+ Following a stroke

Types of Epilepsy

Epilepsy may be generalized or localized (only one part of body or limb is affected), 'Grand-mal' (the classical type of generalized epilepsy) or petit-mal (described below) It can also be classified according to part of brain affected like--Frontal lobe, temporal lobe, occipital lobe etc.

Petit mal Epilepsy

This is also called 'absent' seizures since it is very short lasting (few seconds to half a minute). But it has all the characteristics of an epileptic attack including brief unconsciousness and a disturbed EEG (electro-encephalogram— measures brain waves like an ECG measures electrical waves from the heart) that remains abnormal even in between attacks. There maybe sudden onset of unconsciousness, interruption of any activity, a blank stare, or a brief upward rotation of the eyes. If the patient is speaking, speech is slowed or interrupted, if walking, he suddenly stops, if eating, the food will stop on its way to the mouth. Usually the patient will be unresponsive when spoken to. But in some cases the attacks are aborted when the patient is spoken to. In most cases the attacks can be brought on by making the patient breathe rapidly for three minutes. Sometimes bright light may induce an attack.

Genetic causes of Epilepsy

there are a few types of epilepsy like 'autosomal dominant nocturnal frontal lobe epilepsy' and epilepsy seen in a disease called 'tuberous sclerosis' that have a definite genetic background.

Evaluation of a case of Epilepsy

Evaluation involves trying to find a cause for the epilepsy –was there a head injury in the recent past, any history of headache, fever, loss of weight, diabetes, severe hypertension worm infestation, genetic disease, electrolyte imbalance etc. Tests for all these will have to be carried out. Special tests can include an EEG, CT scan, MRI, SPECT (single photon emission computed tomography), PET (positron emission tomography), MEG (magneto encephalography, brain mapping with electro - corticography etc.

Management of Epilepsy

If an underlying cause is found, taking care of this problem can even *cure* epilepsy. But in many cases, no apparent cause is found even after detailed blood examination, CT or MRI scans of the brain or EEG. For these cases, there are good medicines available to prevent attacks, which should be continued for at least three to five years under medical supervision, and *never* stopped suddenly. Some patients may have to take medication life long. There are many drugs available for treatment of epilepsy, but it is difficult to achieve a balance between effective treatment and no side-effects. In many cases multiple drugs have to be used in lower doses to avoid side-effects. Drug levels in the blood should be checked intermittently to ensure that the dose is correct.

There are also some important dos & don'ts regarding epilepsy that the care-takers of patients should be aware of -

+ If the patient is seated while suffering from the attack, ease him into a lying posture & make sure there are no objects nearby which can cause injury to him.

+ Turn the patient on his stomach & the head to one side for saliva to flow out & also raise his feet by placing on some pillows.

+ Remove any loose objects from the patient's mouth including dentures, if easily possible & remove eyeglasses.

+ Don't crowd around the patient, or try any drastic measures, as most attacks are self-limiting.

+ If the mouth can be opened easily then put a spoon rolled in thick cloth, to prevent tongue bite

+ Do not restrain the patient in anyway.

+ Loosen any tight clothing.

+ Call a doctor or an ambulance only if the attack does not stop.

Surgery for Epilepsy

Resecting tumours or other growths, and repairing vascular malformations are the commonest curative surgeries. Palliative surgery involves procedures that will reduce the frequency and severity of attacks. 'Callostomy' (cutting the corpus callosum that acts as a bridge between the two sides of the brain) can prevent epilepsy from becoming generalised and affecting the whole body. 'Multiple subpial transections' is a similar kind of surgery. In extremely severe cases, half or part of one side of the brain is removed, called 'hemisherectomy'.But this can result in paralysis of the opposite side of the body. 'Gamma knife' surgery is a less invasive form of surgery especially preferred for the brain.

Other Non-surgical Procedures

'Vagus nerve stimulation' –an implant is placed in the chest that connects to the vagus nerve in the neck. The nerve is stimulated at pre-set intervals and intensity, to abort epileptic attacks.

Deep brain stimulation—it is similar to the procedure above, except the device is connected deep into the brain to an area called 'anterior nucleus of thalamus' to abort attacks.

Responsive neurostimulator system—here the device is implanted into the brain at the point or focus from which the epilepsy is originating. As soon as the device detects abnormal charges, it delivers an electrical current into the surrounding area through electrodes placed there, thus aborting the attack.

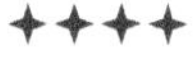

19

Cancer Prevention and Cure

A lot of time and resource is utilised in educating the public about heart disease, but another very important problem i.e. cancer, which is also preventable, with a promise of good outcome if detected early, is largely ignored. Let us attempt to correct this deficiency.

First of all, we must understand that *cancer can be cured if detected early*, and with improvements in investigative techniques and newer medical, surgical and radiation therapies, we can be more optimistic about the results. So let us use every means at our disposal to catch it 'young' and try to eradicate it before it spreads.

Now, how can we help in early detection of cancer? We must look out for the three changes i.e.,

Any change in **Complaints**

Any change in **Look**

Any change in **Feel.**

Change in Complaints

Is there any new and persistent complaint like – persistent pain, vomiting, acidity, diarrhoea, constipation, discharge, bleeding etc. in and from any part of the body?

Change in Look

Have you noticed any new lump, bulge, discolouration or asymmetry in any part of the body? Look out for any change especially in look of moles.

Change in Feel

Can you feel any new lump, hardness, change in texture, on any part of your body or change in any pre-existing lump? -- If you notice any of these *changes*, immediately inform your doctor about them.

Also go in for yearly check-ups with special emphasis on detection of cancer of breast, uterus, and cervix if female, and prostate and testes if male. Incidentally a blood test called PSA (prostate specific antigen) can be used for screening of prostate cancer and mammography (a specialized X-ray of breast) for breast cancer screening. Tobacco chewers should especially look out for white patches on cheeks, and smokers should go in for yearly x-rays of the chest.

Besides early detection, we can also prevent cancer, by proper lifestyle, diet and exercise. Here, more than in any other disease, diet, which is high in fibre content (plenty of vegetables and fruits) and low in fat, is very important as is exercise and prevention of obesity.

Checklist of Carcinogens (things which can cause Cancer)

1. Tobacco chewing - Cancer of mouth and upper gastrointestinal tract.

2. Smoking - Cancer of lungs, bladder, kidney, upper gastrointestinal tract.

3. Alcohol - Cancer of mouth and upper gastrointestinal tract.

4. Obesity - normally associated with hormonal changes and with increased susceptibility to cancer of breast, uterus, cervix, prostate etc.

5. Sexual activity - increased sexual activity especially with diverse partners and unprotected sex, leads to risk of contracting infections with HIV virus (AIDS) and HPV virus (human papilloma virus) – both of which can cause cancer.

6. Moles, Warts and other benign growths may become cancerous.

7. Food preservatives, artificial colourants, reusing oil, charred food (generates carcinogen), out-dated tinned foods etc.

8. Radiation including x–rays - avoid unnecessary x–rays, as your exposure to radiation will keep adding up and chances of cancer increase.

9. Toxic fumes & Gases - from traffic and other sources.

10. UV and Microwaves – too much sunlight, cellular-phones, computers, and microwave ovens.

11. Chemical Fertilisers and Pesticides.

12. Plastic and Polythene - avoid buying moist edibles in thin plastic bags.

13. Stress- Personalities who are not able to withstand stress are also those who are prone to cancer.

Checklist of things which can prevent cancer:

1. Diet- Take plenty of assorted fruits vegetables and nuts

    ✦ Wash vegetables and fruits in running water and add potassium permanganate in final rinse to remove excessive pesticides and fertilisers.

+ Use fresh oil, avoid deep frying & charring of food.

+ Avoid tinned and preserved foods.

+ Avoid foods which can cause hyperacidity – in the long term ulcers may turn cancerous.

2   Avoid tobacco, smoking, alcohol.

3   Get warts and other benign growths attended to or followed up regularly.

4   Keep weight under control, exercise regularly.

6   Go in for yearly check-ups.

7   Learn to do breast self examination.

8   Look out for any change in your body.

9   Avoid stress or learn to control it.

10   Eat out rarely, if at all.

11   Avoid unsafe sex.

12   Utilise sun protection measures in bright sunlight - dark glasses, hats, creams Minimise your use of cell phones, microwave ovens & *wear U.V. filter glasses, while operating computers.*

Management of Cancer

As with other diseases, rapid strides have been made in the management of cancer. Previously we knew of only three methods of treatment. : -

1.   Surgery -by cutting off the growth.

2.   Radiotherapy – using radiation to burn the cancer.

3.   Chemotherapy – use of drugs to kill cancer cells.

Now we have newer methods of treatment like -

1.   **Radio or Stereotactic Surgery**- Here a three-dimensional

radio beam using a special head frame is directed at the tumour and the cancer is destroyed. It is ideal for brain tumours, and since no knife is used directly on the brain, chances of damage to surrounding healthy cells are minimal. Hospital stay is also cut down.

2. **Laser Surgery** - surgical resection using laser—more precise, and less blood loss.

3. **C R Y O Surgery** - especially for liver cancer. Here a hollow tube is introduced into the tumour and liquid nitrogen at minus 190° is poured in. The resulting ice ball destroys the tumour.

4. **Genetic Therapy** - for certain hereditary tumours, genetic mapping is done, the defective gene removed. & healthy gene introduced to prevent cancer from occurring.

5. **Bone marrow transplantation** – There are many blood cancers which can be treated by destroying the bone marrow (which produces blood cells) with radiation, and then after starting anti- rejection drugs, replacing with marrow from a well-matched donor. In many cases, cure can be achieved.

6. **Cord blood transplantation** - Umbilical cord that connects the baby to the mother during pregnancy contains stem cells (which produce normal blood cells like bone marrow.) Here even without 100% matching, chances of rejection are less, so we should learn to preserve this useful biological waste

7. **Targeted drug therapy** - for liver cancer. Here a tube is passed directly into the liver artery, and the anti-cancer drug is delivered so that the generalised toxic effect of oral medication is avoided.

8. **Immunotherapy** - here cancer cells (antigens) are

removed and antibodies grown against them outside the body. These antibodies when introduced, fight against the cancer cells, and destroy them.

9. **Proton and Photon** - therapy especially for cancer prostrate .

10. **Psychotherapy** is also needed to boost the morale, and not give in as miracles can always happen.

11. **Newer Drugs** and methods for managing cancer pain.

With all these advances in managing cancer, it may not remain the nightmare that it was till recently.

So let your eyes and fingers act as watch dogs, while you look out for any *changes* in your body, and catch that crab before it claws its way all over you!

Breast Examination-

Cancer of breast is difficult to detect, and since it is very important that it be detected early, proper self-examination of breasts must be learnt. Ideally examination should be done every month, after forty. You should do it immediately after periods, or on the first day of the month, if menopausal.

What you should look for: - - Is there any change in the breasts since you last saw them? Is there any new asymmetry? Do the nipples look indented, or inverted? Is there any dimpling or roughening (orange peel look) anywhere on the breasts? Is there any bulge or change in contour? (You may appreciate this better by raising your hands, above your head) Look out for any changes in the armpits also.

Palpation (feeling)

First feel the nipples – is there any *change* in feel or *any discharge on squeezing?*

If your breasts are pendulous and big, support one breast with your left hand. (pictures below) Now place four fingers of right hand (except thumb) on the breasts and using their flat surfaces, firmly pressed on breast, move them around, starting from 12 0'clock position, and going round the clock, till 11 0 'clock position. Try to discern any lump between the flat surfaces of fingers of right hand, and the chest wall. If you feel something, try to roll it between fingers and chest wall - if it rolls, it is a lump. There may be patches of thickened breast tissue, which you will learn to appreciate and ignore *especially in the lower inner part of breast.* When you have finished examining one breast, switch over to the other, and repeat the process. Finally look out for palpable glands in both the armpits and above the collarbones. The pictures below will help you to understand the correct method of examination.

If thinly built, you can examine the breast without support of the other hand. Besides self-examination, you should have a yearly check-up with your family physician (six monthly in high risk cases), and mammography as advised by your physician. *If you have history of breast cancer in the family, are unmarried, obese or married with only one or two children, or have not breast-fed your children, or taking hormonal replacement therapy, you are at a higher risk than the general population.*

Breast Self Examination

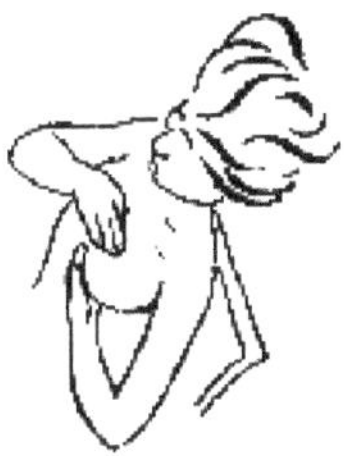

Examine with support of opposite hand if the breast is heavy

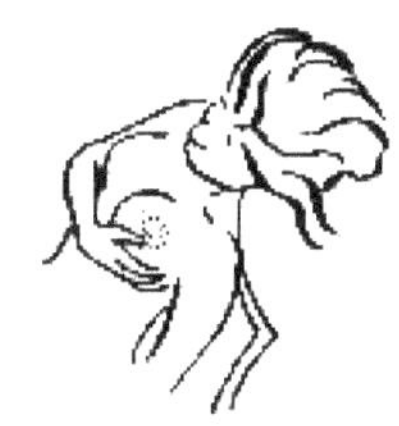

Look for any rough spot on skin (like an orange peel)

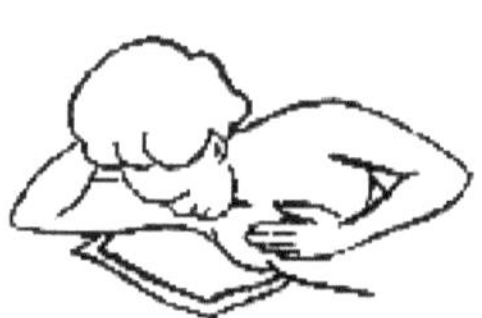

Lie down on your bed, put a pillow or
bath towel under your left shoulder,
& your left hand under your head,
and now examine the breast.

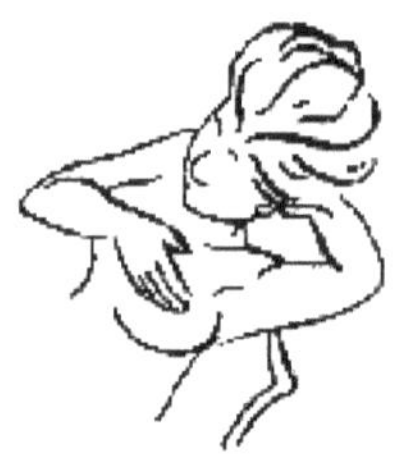

Use the four fingers
flattened on the
breast and roll
against chest

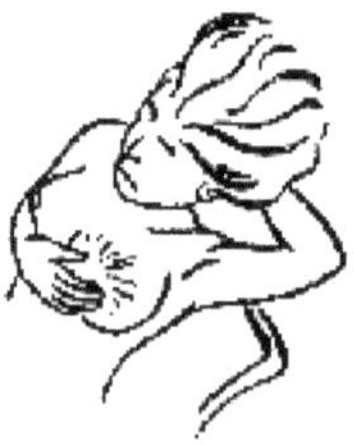

Always examine the breast
in a clockwise manner

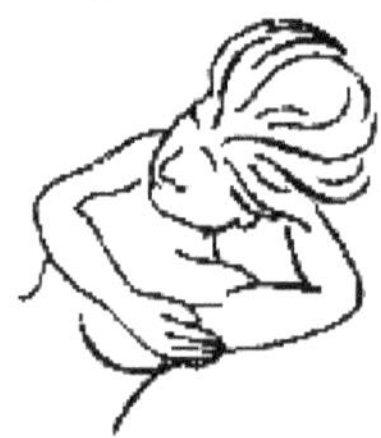

Now feel under your
armpits.

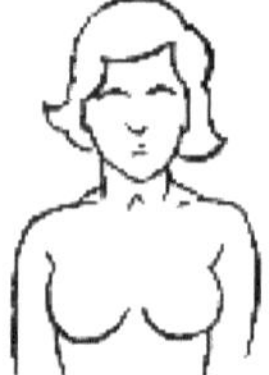

Sit or stand in front of the mirror,
arms relaxed at your sides, & look
for any changes in the breasts.

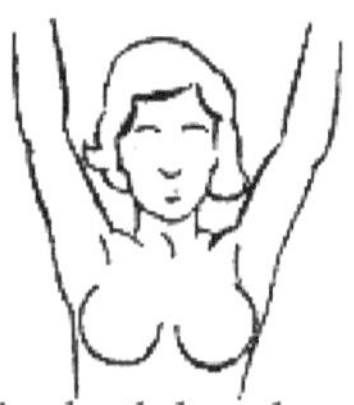

Raise both hands over
your head & look for
the same things.

Examination of the
breast in the shower: -
wet surface permits e asy
feeling.

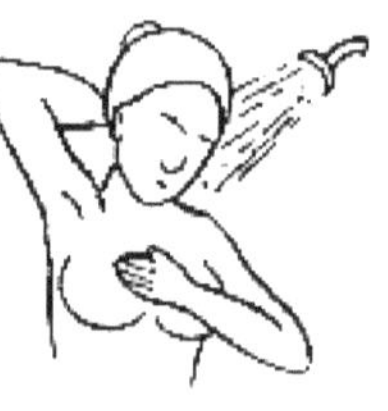

Self-examination in Males

Men must learn to look out for any changes in their testes and any new urinary problems which may indicate testicular or prostatic cancer.

They must also examine their mouths for any changes if they are tobacco chewers and report to their doctors immediately if there is any non responding cough especially if accompanied by blood in the sputum if they are smokers.

Biopsy: Biopsy is a procedure where a piece of tissue is cut from a superficial or deep growth, which is then sliced and examined under the microscope for any cancerous changes.

FNAC (Fine needle aspiration cytology) here, a syringe and needle are used to suck out some tissue from a superficial growth, which is then examined under a microscope for any changes.

PAP Smear: In this procedure, the cells shed by the uterus are collected, smeared on a slide and examined for any cancerous or even pre- cancerous changes.

Case Study:

While at medical college, we saw a lady with advanced cancer (it had spread all over the body including the skeletal system). The treating consultant knew nothing could be done and advised her to go on a pilgrimage. The old lady did just that and believe it or not, this is a documented case where her x-rays came back to normal. Faith healing? More likely the lady's immunity had been stimulated leading to a cure.

✦✦✦✦

20

Sexual Dysfunction

No book on forty plus can be complete without a chapter on sexual disorders. As we grow older, since our hormonal levels reduce, desire for sex and performance are bound to decrease. Reduced desire should be compensated by being more loving and caring and sharing each other's joys and problems and attempts should be made to keep oneself attractive and trim. Exercise, like in other problems, helps here too. Smoking, tobacco chewing, intake of alcoholic drinks should be avoided, and anything which leads to bad breath like raw onion, garlic, indigestion and oral infections should be taken care of. Anxiety and depression can lead to sexual dysfunction, and can be helped by psychological counseling or mild medication.

Common problems encountered can be—

In Women:

Dryness of Vagina	Reduced Desire
Pain during Sexual Act	Orgasmic Disorder

Non hormonal or phyto-oestrogens, local lubricating creams, and oestrogen creams may be used.

Food sources of Phyto-oestrogens or Isoflavones are -

Carrots	Tomato	Wheat
Beetroot	Apple	Yam

Pumpkin	Plum	Saunf
Potato	Papaya	(fennel seeds)
Bengal gram	Pomegranate	Black pepper
Cucumber	Garlic	Oats
Dates	Brinjal (Egg-plant)	Cherries
Soya	Jeera (Cumin)	Peas
Lin-Seed (Red clover)	Par-boiled rice	Barley

Men : Erectile dysfunction- it is the medical term for impotence, or the inability to maintain an erection during intercourse. It can be due to vascular, neurological, endocrinal or kidney-disease, certain drugs and addictions, psychological, and some local causes. According to one study, over 47 million men are afflicted with this problem and after forty 5 – 15 % of men will have suffered from it.

1. Vascular - due to ischaemic heart disease, hypertension, atherosclerotic heart disease, peripheral vessel disease.

2. Neurological-diseases of spine or peripheral nerves.

3. Endocrinal causes like diabetes, hypothyroidism, hypopituitarism, and hyper-prolactinaemia.

4. Kidney diseases –kidney failure or dialysis.

5. Psychological - misconceptions about sex, poor self-esteem, marital discord, anxiety or depression.

6. Local Causes - injury, deformities, infections, or tumors.

7. Addictions like alcohol, or tobacco.

8. Drugs like those used for blood pressure, psychosis, depression, irregularity in pulse, lowering of lipids, epilepsy and hyper acidity. Others are anti- inflammatory drugs, steroids and oral contraceptive pills.

No qualified Sexologist will advise medication in the preliminary stages and proper counseling, behavioral and other techniques should correct most problems. Quacks should not be consulted as their medications may be harmful and effects unpredictable.

Discuss with your doctor, if any medication you are taking is the cause of your problem, and if substitutes can be prescribed (in both sexes).

Treatment of erectile dysfunction-

1. Drugs like sildenafil, (viagra), phentolamine, apomorphine, etc.
2. Local creams.
3. Local injections.
4. Prosthetic devices (to help in maintaining erection).
5. Surgery for correcting deformities.
6. Hormone replacement therapy.
7. Vacuum devices.

Viagra - acts by increasing blood supply to penile tissue. It starts acting in 60 minutes and effect lasts for four-six hours. It works in 70% of cases, but people with hypertension, and especially those taking nitrate drugs, should be very cautious as it can cause fall in blood pressure. It can also cause some visual changes, & should not be used in those with sluggish liver & kidney functions. Many medications can increase the action of Viagra such as - erythromycin, antacids, some diuretics, rifampicin (for T. B), and some medicines for B.P., & diabetes- beta blockers, alpha blockers, calcium channel blockers, protease inhibitors (HIV medicines) tolbutamide etc. and the results may be unpredictable.

Dose - 25-50 milligrams once a day, 1-4 hours before intercourse.

   + Use with caution- in elderly.
   + Contraindications (not to be used).
   + Men suffering from ischaemic heart disease.
   + Patients on nitrates.

- ✦ Recent stroke.
- ✦ Severe liver disease.
- ✦ Severe kidney problem.
- ✦ Retinal problems.
- ✦ Children.

Dapoxetine

This is another FDA approved drug for premature ejaculation in men.

Dose – one tablet of 30milligrams, 1-3 hours before intercourse only once in 24 hours.

Common side effects are headache, dizziness, nausea, and diarrhea.

In less than 10% there can be dryness of mouth, stomach pain, anxiety, weakness, tremors, sweating and stuffy nose.

Rarely there can be loss of sexual drive, high blood pressure, fainting when standing up, and irregular heart rate.

Disadvantages of currently available methods of treatments-

1. Long term treatment is required
2. Side effects of drugs, sometimes-serious ones.
3. Unpredictable results.
4. Most treatments are expensive.
5. Some are still in the experimental stage.

So, if you want to go in for treatment, go to only a qualified sexologist with some experience, & try to understand all the consequences, before starting any therapy.

Reference - IJIM SPECIAL ISSUE ISSN O971-2925.

✦✦✦✦

21

Menopause, Uterus and Prostate

"Today is the first day of the rest of your life"
- Dale Carnegie

"Meno " means month, and *"Pause"* means to halt - menopause thus means stoppage of monthly cycles. It is a three to five year period during which ovarian functions begin to decline and finally stop. Besides natural menopause, ovarian functions can decline in patients who have had their uterus and ovaries removed or taken radiotherapy for cancer.

There are so many misconceptions about menopause that all of us expect to have some problems as we approach that dreaded age of forty-five. It is not necessary that everyone will have problems, and minor ones should be taken in stride and considered normal. Some patients may have severe complaints transiently, and only a minority of women have persistent problems, which need treatment. Common complaints can be hot flushes, night sweats, palpitations, (being conscious of one's heart beats), increased risk of urinary infection, dryness and sagging of skin and vagina, bone thinning, irritability, fatigue and sometimes depression. *Menopause is a natural condition and must be treated as such.* If you keep busy, eat nutritious food, exercise regularly, and have a positive attitude, things will normally settle down after some time, and you will hardly realize that you have reached menopause.

One thing you must understand is that oestrogen (a female hormone) protects women from atherosclerosis and keeps the bones strong, and after menopause as the protective effect of this hormone is lost they may become prone to hypertension, heart disease and osteoporosis (bone softening). Greater stress has to be laid on good calcium –rich diets-(discussed in chapter on Nutrition) as also low fat and low salt food, with plenty of weight bearing exercises during menopausal age to offset these problems

Soya- all peri- menopausal women should be encouraged to consume Soya and its products in some form or the other, since it contains phyto oestrogens (see previous chapter for other sources of phyto-oestrogens) which act like oestrogen. Vitamin E also helps in hot flushes.

Hot Flushes and Night Sweats- menopausal women may get hot flushes. This is because the skin temperature goes up for five to six minutes intermittently, due to lack of oestrogen which makes women wake up suddenly at night sweating profusely, leaving them tired & drained out the next day.

H R T - You must have heard about 'hormonal replacement therapy'. This is supplementing oestrogen from outside to take care of the reduced secretion in the body.

Merits : As already mentioned, oestrogen helps in keeping skin supple, vagina moist, eliminates mood swings, helps retain sexual function, slows down atheroselerosis, and keeps bones strong. Since the average woman will live 20-30 years after menopause, these problems will be less if she takes HRT.

Demerits: HRT can increase risk of uterine and breast cancer although giving natural as opposed to synthetic oestrogen, and combining with another hormone called Progesterone can lower incidence of uterine cancer,. If HRT is taken, monthly self-breast examination and 6 monthly examinations by a doctor is a must as also frequent mammographies & pap smears, to detect any cancer. It also doubles the risk of gall bladder problems, vaginal bleeding, breast tenderness, nausea, bloating due to, fluid retention, liver problems, headache & migraine, blood clots, changes in shape of eyes, dizziness & depression.

Contra indications to HRT

There are certain conditions where HRT, should not be taken, for e.g.-

+ Undiagnosed vaginal bleeding
+ Genetic predisposition to uterine or breast cancer
+ Thromboembolic disease (block in vessels)
+ History of endometriosis (uterine inner lining grows inwards into muscles)
+ Liver and gall bladder disease
+ Menstrual migraine (those patients who used to get headache during periods)

Other drugs that act like oestrogen

Tibolone—it is a synthetic steroid which has the effects of all three hormones secreted by the ovaries—oestrogen, progesterone and testosterone. It helps in hot flushes and also decreased libido. It does not stimulate tissues of the uterus like HRT does, so it is superior.

Use with caution—

+ Kidney disease
+ Migraine
+ Epilepsy
+ High cholesterol

Not to be used-

+ History of breast cancer
+ Heart attacks
+ Stroke
+ Liver problems
+ Tibolone can react with anti-coagulant drugs (warfarin),
  some drugs used for tuberculosis and epilepsy. Some
  women can get masculinising side effects like greasy skin
  and abnormal hair growth.

Raloxifene

This is an oral selective oestrogen receptor modulator (SERM)
that has the beneficial effect that oestrogen has on strengthening
bone, and anti oestrogen action on breast and uterus that
prevents cancer of these organs. It is thus extremely useful in
post menopausal women with osteoporosis, especially those at
risk of breast cancer or those who have already suffered from it.
Only major side effect is it increases tendency towards
thrombosis all over the body, including the retina. This can lead
to increased incidence of stroke. Other side effects include,
swelling in legs, breathlessness, blurring of vision.

You can discuss all this with your doctor and take a decision,
whether to take HRT, Tibolone, or Raloxifene and for how long,
after carefully weighing the merits and demerits.

Finally I would like to re-emphasize that menopause *is not a
disease* and as far as possible no medications should be taken
unless your complaints are very severe. There is no need to fear
its approach and get depressed when it does, and now that you
are aware of the advantages of good nutrition and exercise, and
hopefully will begin to implement them, chances are, you will
have an easy transitional phase. Now let us try to understand
some common surgical conditions and procedures to do with the

reproductive system.

Hysterectomy – (Removal of Uterus)

Uterus can be removed under the following conditions –

1. Severe bleeding not controlled by maximal medical effort
2. Cancer of reproductive organs
3. Growths like fibroids if too many or too big
4. Prolapse (descent of uterus from its position)
5. An abnormal PAP smear – (explained later)

Normally when uterus is removed, the ovaries are left intact since they produce useful female hormones, which also help your heart and bones; but if there is cancer, or if the patient is nearing menopause, then ovaries are also removed.

"**Papanicoleau or Pap Smear**" – a routine test in which we collect the uterine cells which are shed outside, on a slide and study them under a microscope looking for any abnormal cells. If there are too many of them, we do a *hysteroscopic biopsy.* Here a fibre optic self-illuminated tube is used to visualise the inside of the uterus, biopsies are taken by the same instrument from suspicious areas; and material is examined under a microscope to confirm any abnormality.

Colposcopy -- Here the lower part of the female reproductive organs are studied under magnification for any problems.

Prolapse - Prolapse is descent of the uterus from its position because of its attachments becoming weak. It can be graded according to degree into four grades.

In grade-I, part of the uterus descends and presses on urinary bladder and /or terminal part of intestines (rectum) and in grade IV, it comes out completely and does not go back. In those with grade III – IV who are otherwise fit, it is better to remove the uterus, and in older patients where major surgery is risky, there is a 'sling' operation where uterus is pulled up and tied.

In grade I and II stages and in younger patients, operation should only be considered if there are complications like recurrent bladder infection (because of pressure on urinary passage) or severe constipation, due to pressure on rectum etc.

UTERUS – front view

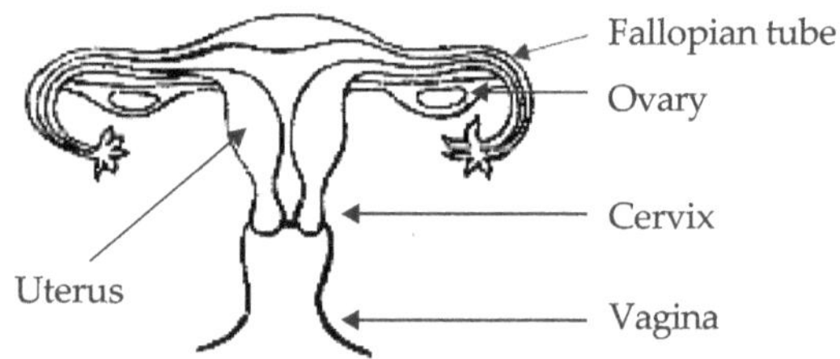

UTERUS – side view

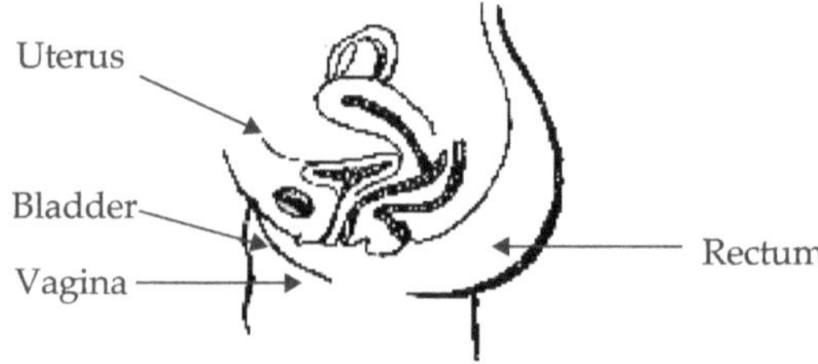

PROSTATE PROBLEMS

When the hair turns grey, the arteries harden and the eye lens becomes opaque, it is also the time when the prostate gland in males begins to enlarge.

What is prostate?

It is a collection of glands situated below the urinary bladder and surrounding the urinary passage. It has a sexual function by contributing a tiny fraction to seminal fluid. It also contracts during intercourse thus preventing retrograde-ejaculation. Prostate enlargement can sometimes turn cancerous, but most cases are non- malignant and are   called BPH or Benign Prostatic Hypertrophy

A patient suffering from BPH may complain of frequency of urination, thinning of stream, dribbling, or sense of incomplete urination, due to compression of urinary passage. If neglected, complications can develop like urine infection, bladder stones, and retention of urine, blood in urine or kidney failure.

Diagnosis is made by the complaints, by examination and by sonography. There are also two blood tests called *PSA* (prostate specific antigen) and *acid phosphatase* which when increased should make us suspect cancerous change. *Urine flow studies* can also be done to assess the exact degree of obstruction.

Management of prostatic enlargement can be by medical or surgical methods. There are now many medicines which help in reducing size of prostate, and prevent further enlargement; but if complications develop, surgery should be resorted to - for e.g., when there is,

1. Significant residual urine in bladder after voiding (more than 100ml)
2. Recurrent urinary infection
3. Blood in urine
4. Change into cancer.
5. Urine flow less than 10ml per second

Types of surgery available are -

T U R P (Trans urethral resection of prostate)

1. Here a self-illuminated tube like instrument is passed into the urine passage and the cutting end of the same instrument is used to remove the prostate. There are no stitches in this procedure and 95% of cases of prostate surgery are done by this method.

2. Surgery by open method, where the abdomen is cut up (the usual method of surgery)

3. By laser.

In conclusion, go in for a check-up with your doctor, and if your prostate is enlarged, do a yearly sonography to assess its size and the amount of residual urine, PSA, acid phosphatase and   urine flow studies if you can afford it. If there are any indicators of immediate surgery (as outlined above) go in for it, otherwise medical management can continue.

PROSTATE GLAND

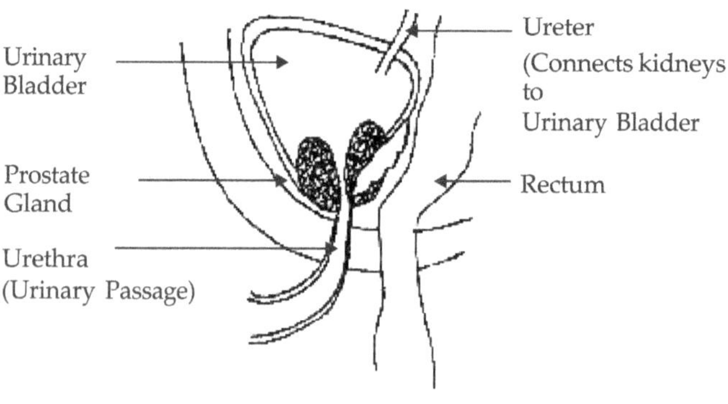

✦ ✦ ✦ ✦

Part – IV

Some useful
Health related
Knowledge

22

Nutrition and Diet

*"Jack sprat ate all the fat, his wife ate all the lean;
And so between the two of them, They licked the platter
clean",*

Great economy, but obviously wrong eating habits on both sides!

"We are what we eat", so the first thing to understand is the dos and don'ts of nutrition. As we grow older we should change our diets both in quality and quantity. High fat and high protein foods like meat, eggs, groundnuts, pistachio, cashew, ghee (clarified butter), butter, cheese, fried foods, cream etc. are not required except in small quantities, after we stop growing; and if we continue to consume them, we will end up growing sideways! We must also cut down on quantity of cereals, and oil, compensating by increasing the intake of more beneficial items like fruits, vegetables and sprouts.

Food should be eaten fresh and warm, avoiding extremes of temperature. Raw items (like salads and fruits) should be eaten within four hours of cutting. Ideally the heaviest meal of the day should be breakfast and the lightest—dinner -

"Breakfast like a Prince

Lunch like a courtier

And sup like a pauper"

Food pyramid should thus look like this:

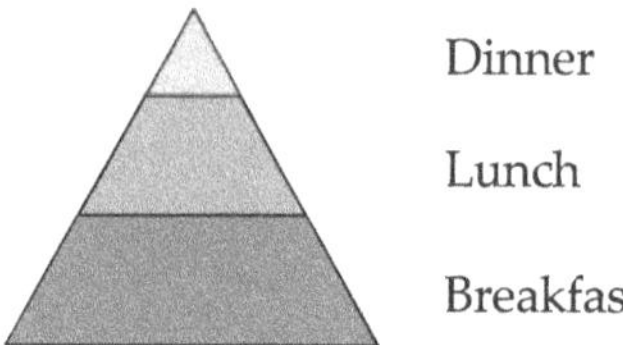

Regularity and proper spacing of meals are also important. Fasting, in a diabetic should be avoided, and feasting? - A big NO for every one.

Now let us understand what the constituents of our food are and a little bit about each of them -

CONSTITUENTS OF FOOD

Carbohydrates : These are our main sources of energy and are provided by - sugar, honey, fruits, certain root vegetables, cereals and dairy products. 60% of our energy requirement should come from this group.

Proteins : Proteins are required for growth and repair. As we grow older, only 20% of our energy requirement should come from proteins. Dairy products, cereals, pulses, nuts and fish are good protein sources. Meat and eggs also contain good quality proteins but their intake should be reduced after twenty-five years of age (white of egg is ok).

Soya is a useful nutritional aid. It has very high and good quality protein content, comparable with non-vegetarian food, without the disadvantages of the latter (high fat, low fibre). Because of high protein content, the stomach takes longer to empty and frequent hunger is avoided. Soya also contains phyto-oestrogens (natural female hormones), which are very useful for women after menopause, and good fats, which help the heart. It can be taken as a drink, as nuggets or chunks in vegetables, as a cereal to mix with wheat flour for making chapattis etc. In short for good nutrition, to reduce weight, to correct lipid imbalance and to avoid menopausal problems, incorporate soya in your diet.

Fats : This is the stored form of energy. During emergency situations, it is converted into easily utilized form. Only 20% of our energy requirement should come from fats, that too mainly unsaturated (Fat or oil which remains liquid at room temperature).

Note: *More about fats in the chapter on atherosclerotic heart disease, and in 'All about oil!'*

Water : Depending on our age, 50 – 70% of our body is composed of water. It is the vehicle which carries nutrition to the cells and toxins out of them; hence eight - ten glasses of water a day is absolutely essential for proper functioning of the body. While a human can survive more than a week without food, a person will die within a few days without water. Physically active individuals generally have more water in their bodies than those who are less physically active. Because they sweat more, active people need to replenish water more often, thus raising their water level. A trained male runner may have up to 71 percent water in his body, while a female gymnast may have 70 percent. Obese individuals, on the other hand, have a lower percentage of water in their bodies (about 48%). You can see from this that physically active people remain as young as children if you use water content of the body as a yardstick. They also have a better muscle mass and calcium content in their bones which we will talk about later. Conversely, a young obese person has the water content of an aged individual! Water balance refers to the balance between the amount of water consumed and the amount of water excreted.

Functions of water

+ The body's water content needs to be constant for its optimal functioning. Cells are bathed in fluids that contain nutrients; they source these nutrients from them. These fluids also carry wastes away from the cells. Water also helps in exchange of salts in and out of cells. Water lubricates joints and acts as shock absorber inside the eyes, brain and spinal cord and the unborn baby inside the uterus.

+ Water also helps the body maintain a constant temperature by acting as a thermostat. When a person is too hot, the body sweats; when sweat evaporates, it lowers the body temperature. Conversely, when the body feels very cold, the skin pores close, we sweat less and heat is conserved inside the body. We also conserve and lose water through our breath and our kidneys. In fact water helps in efficient functioning of kidneys.

+ Water also helps in keeping our skin supple and healthy.

Now that you've understood its importance, make sure you drink 8-10 glasses of water; drink this as water itself or in the form of milk, buttermilk, soups, beverages, etc.

Do not drink water with food; it will dilute the digestive enzymes from the mouth.

Alcohol, tea and coffee have diuretic effects (cause increased urination), so they are not good substitutes for water.

Minerals and vitamins : These are required in minute quantities but perform essential functions. They are present in cereals, pulses, meat and dairy products also, but mainly in fruits and vegetables. *500grams each of mi/ed fruits and vegetables divided into 2-3 helpings a day provide enough minerals and vitamins.*

Table showing Recommended daily allowance (RDA) in adults

Total Fat65 g Saturated Fatty Acids 20 g Cholesterol 300 mg Sodium 2300 mg Potassium 4700 mg Total Carbohydrate 300 g Fiber 25 g Protein 50 g For vitamins and minerals, the RDA are given in the following table

Nutrient RDI

Vitamin A	5000	IU
Vitamin	C60	mg
Calcium	1000	mg
Iron	18	mg
Vitamin	D400	IU
Vitamin	E30	IU
Vitamin	K80	µg
Thiamin	1.5	mg
Riboflavin	1.7	mg
Niacin	20	mg
Vitamin	B62	mg
Folate	400	µg
Vitamin	B126	µg
Biotin	300	µg
Pantothenic acid	10	mg
Phosphorus	1000	mg
Iodine	150	µg
Magnesium	400	mg
Zinc	15	mg
Selenium	70	µg
Copper	2	mg
Manganese	2	mg
Chromium	120	µg

| Molybdenum | 75 | µg |
| Chloride | 3400 | mg |

Vitamins can be fat soluble (which bind to fat in the body and are stored) OR water soluble, excess of which is thrown out in the urine by the kidneys.

Fat soluble vitamins are A, D, E and K

Vitamin A is available as itself (called *retinol*) or as a Pro vitamin called *Beta-carotene.*

Retinol is present in animal foods like milk and its products, eggs, meat and fish.

Beta Carotene is present in green leafy vegetables and yellow fruits and vegetables like carrots, papaya, mango etc. Beta Carotenes have excellent anti- oxidant effects (explained later)

35 grams of dark, green leafy vegetables or 100 grams of yellow fruit or a small helping of fish liver, or a glass of milk are enough to supply daily requirement of Beta carotene.

Prolonged high temperature cooking, exposure to high intensity light or rancidity (rotting) of food, destroys the vitamin, but frozen foods retain their vitamin A content for long.

Uses: Vitamin A is required for good eyesight in dark, maintaining supple skin, integrity of all linings in body, and healthy growth of embryo (baby inside the womb).

Vitamin D

Vitamin D increases calcium and phosphorus absorption from the intestines and thus stimulates bone formation. Recently there have been some studies that indicate that it may protect us from cancer. It is available to us as Pro- vitamin or inactive form in skin, and as active form from food. Inactive form from the skin is converted to active form on exposure to sunlight, so exposure to sunlight is very important and even the aged should be encouraged to sit out in the sun at least for an hour everyday, to convert their inactive vitamin D into the active form.

Active vitamin D is present in milk and its products, fish liver, and yeast. Inactive vitamin D from the skin is very efficiently and slowly converted into active vitamin D in the liver, as it is available only in small amounts at a time. But active vitamin D from food is presented rapidly to the liver, and the liver degrades most of it to prevent toxic accumulation in the body. Thus very little is available to the body for use. So, it is preferable to source your vitamin D by getting your body to convert the inactive form in your skin to active vitamin-D, as its availability is better. What I am trying to say is *go out and elercise in the sunlight!*

The ability to absorb and synthesize vitamin D decreases with age. Supplementation with calcium and Vitamin D may be required in growing children, pregnant women and the old.

Dietary sources of active vitamin D are milk and its products, fish liver and yeast.

Uses: It is needed for healthy bones, teeth and muscles and for proper utilisation of phosphorous and calcium.

Vitamin E - is present in Soya bean, wheat germ, rice germ and lettuce leaves. It is required for proper functioning of reproductive organs, nervous system and vascular system. It is a good anti-oxidant.

Vitamin K - 50% of vitamin K is synthesised in the intestinal tract by bacteria, which are normally residing there in harmony with the body (all bacteria are therefore not bad!). It is also present in most green vegetables.

Uses: It is required for preventing bleeding by helping in the formation of *blood clot* (plug.)

Anti-oxidants - During normal cellular activity, certain 'free radicals' are released. These are elements with one of their electrons missing. In trying to retrieve their 'lost electron' these radicals go berserk, turning into 'rogue elements' and destroying cells in their path. These free radicals may be 'free oxygen', hydroxyl ions, super oxide dysmutase etc. Unless they are 'quenched' or destroyed, they can lead to extensive damage. These quenchers are called "anti-oxidants". Examples are – vitamin C, vitamin E, B-carotene, selenium etc., which by their 'anti-oxidant' action prevent chronic diseases.

Water Soluble Vitamins

These are B complex and Vitamin C.

B Complex – These are of various types clubbed under an umbrella of 'B Complex'

They are present in various vegetables, fruits, milk, yeast, legumes (peas, beans etc.) peanuts, pulses, meat and eggs.

Uses: They are needed for nerve functions, carbohydrate breakdown, healthy body linings and formation of blood and other cells.

Folic acid- this is an important water soluble vitamin.

There is a chemical in the blood called homocysteine. It is a breakdown product of certain proteins in the body. This chemical damages blood vessels and increases the stickiness of blood, which means it brings cells together. Now we all know that anything which increases stickiness of blood will hasten the process of atherosclerosis or hardening and narrowing of blood vessels, that is responsible for hypertension, heart and paralytic attacks. Folic acid is a vitamin that brings down homocysteine levels, and therefore reduces stickiness of blood, so it is a good idea to get enough of it from our diet. Folic acid is also required for cell growth especially red blood cells. Along with Vitamin B-12, it therefore prevents a type of anaemia called megaloblastic anaemia. Since it is required for cell-growth, it has a special role to play in the first three months of pregnancy, as there is maximum cell growth and multiplication of the foetus (baby), inside the uterus during this period. Now what are the rich sources of folic acid? These are---*tomatoes, green peas, spinach, ladies finger, lentils and black eyed peas.* So make sure you eat plenty of these if you want your cells to multiply in a healthy way and prevent stickiness of blood.

Vitamin B-12

We have already spoken of its importance in prevention of anaemia. It is also required for proper functioning of nerves, and if its levels are low, we can have *neuropathy* ---leading to sensation of tingling and numbness, and also general weakness. All patients of anaemia should have their vitamin B-12 levels checked, especially if they are vegetarians--- because this vitamin is deficient in a vegetarian diet. But luckily dairy products like milk, curd, cheese, butter, ghee (clarified butter) etc. are rich sources. Vegetarians should make sure they consume at least three cups a day of milk and three cups of curd or 3 glasses of buttermilk, and some paneer (cottage cheese), to get enough of this vitamin.

Vitamin C is present in sour fruits like orange, lemons, avla (Indian gooseberry) tomatoes and also in potatoes and green vegetables.

Uses: It prevents bleeding, helps in blood formation, promotes wound healing and assists in bone and cartilage growth.

Calcium - Milk, milk products, green leafy vegetables, ragi (millet) and other cereals are good sources of calcium. Growing children, post menopausal women and both sexes above sixty five years of age require supplements.

Uses: It is required for healthy bones and teeth, nerve and muscle functions and helps in blood clotting.

On an average, only 25-30% of the calcium we consume is absorbed. Since it is a very important mineral especially for ladies, and for all old people, I am going to discuss it in detail. Calcium from milk source is 100% absorbed and from green leafy vegetables very poorly absorbed because of the presence of phosphates and oxalates. Similarly calcium from cereals is also poorly absorbed, because of the presence of phytates. Ragi (makra/ nachni/ Indian Millet) is one of the richest sources of calcium, and polished rice one of the poorest. Absorption of calcium is increased in the presence of parathormone, a hormone secreted from the parathyroid glands in the neck, vitamin D and a protein rich diet. Calcitonin, another hormone secreted from thyroid glands in the neck, acts in the opposite direction by increasing *calcium loss* through the kidneys.

Calcium Requirement

Age	Required Calcium In Milligrams Per Day
Birth-6 Months	400
6 Months To 1yr	600
1 Yr –10 Yrs	800-1200
25-50 Yrs (Men and Women)	1000
51-64 Yrs (Men and Women on ERT)*	1000
51+ (Women not on ERT)	1500
65+	1500

Source-National Institute of Health India

***ERT- Estrogen Replacement Therapy**

If you want to avoid taking calcium supplements, I have created a table to show you how it can be done -

**Table Showing Calcium Content Of Easily
Absorbable Vegetarian Sources Of Calcium**

Food item	Amount	Calcium content
Milk	300 ml. (2 cups)	240 mgs.
Curds	300 ml. (2 cups)	240 mgs.
Pulses	200 ml. (2 cups)	360 mgs.
Sprouts	50 mgs. (1/2 cup)	080 mgs.
Soya	50 mgs. (1/2 cup)	120 mgs.
Ragi(millet)	50 mgs. (1/2 cup)	165 mgs.
Skimmed milk powder	15 gms. (3 tea- spoons)	225 mgs.
	Total	**1430 mgs**

So if we consume the food items shown above in the amounts specified, we will be taking in 1430 milligrams of calcium a day.

Remaining 70 milligrams (to give us a maximum of 1500 mgs.) can easily be obtained from fruits, cereals and vegetables. Actually cereals, vegetables and fruits will provide at least 1000milligrams of calcium, and even if 30% is absorbed, we will get 300 milligrams, and skimmed milk powder can be excluded from the table.

Calcium supplements

Supplemental calcium reduces bone loss in older women, especially in those who have very low dietary calcium intakes. It is also advised in growing children, pregnancy and lactation. All calcium supplements irrespective of the compound are poorly absorbed and can cause constipation and gastric irritation except for ionic calcium that is better absorbed and causes fewer problems. Understand your need and take supplements according to your doctor's advice. Excessive calcium can interfere with absorption of phosphorus (which is also useful in preventing osteoporosis) from the intestines.

Iron - Rich sources of iron are green vegetables, dates, gur, (unrefined cane sugar) meat, bananas, apples, prunes, raisins, figs,dates,and egg yolk. Cooking in iron pots also increases iron content of food.

Vitamin C rich foods help in iron absorption, like---tomatoes, lemon, orange, amla(Indian gooseberry).

Beta carotene rich foods also aid absorption, like—all red and yellow fruits and vegetables.

Antacids and calcium supplements interfere with absorption of iron and should not be taken along with iron supplements.

Uses: Iron is required for the formation of blood.

Like calcium iron is a very important mineral, and I'm going to discuss it in detail. Every cell in the body has iron, and it is present in the body in three forms -

+ Present as haem - in haemoglobin (in blood), myoglobin (in muscles), and also as a constituent of various enzymes.
+ Present as protein bound form as - transferrin (the transport form of iron.)
+ Present as the stored form of iron called - haemosiderin and ferritin.

This knowledge is very important because in iron deficiency it is not enough to give iron till haemoglobin comes to normal; it is important to replenish the stores also (about 30 % extra) - otherwise there will be a relapse of anaemia. There is a test called *serum ferritin* that gives us an indication of the amount of stored iron.

What is the daily requirement of iron?

Children	8-18mg
Men	10-15mg
Women	15-20mg.
Pregnanc and lactation	20-25mg.

Iron facts -

✦ Iron from vegetarian sources is poorly absorbed. (1-6%) because of the presence of phytates.

✦ Iron from non-vegetarian sources is better absorbed- around 10%. Egg yolk, meat and fish are good sources especially liver, heart and crabs. However iron from eggs is poorly absorbed because of presence of phosphates. Lack of vitamin C also interferes with iron absorption from non vegetarian sources.

✦ *Ferrous* salts are more easily absorbed. *Ferric* salts have to be first converted into ferrous form to be absorbed.

✦ Acid from the stomach is *essential* to ionise iron from food to make it absorbable. Acid suppressing drugs may therefore interfere with its absorption. But in some patients who have severe gastric irritation due to iron, we may have to give antacids along or before iron preparations.

- ✦ Vitamin C and proteins in food help in converting ferric into ferrous form.
- ✦ Food interferes with iron absorption but in some patients who cannot tolerate iron; it has to be given with or after food.
- ✦ Iron absorption is also reduced in conditions of diarrhoea and conditions of malabsorption.
- ✦ Iron absorption rises proportionately to the severity of anaemia. Thus haemoglobin levels will rise faster in a patient whose level is only 5g% as compared to one in whom it is 10g%.
- ✦ Iron is also available to the body from the destruction of ageing red blood cells.
- ✦ Iron is lost from the body in stools, urine, sweat and menstrual fluid. Out of these, loss in sweat can be excessive in tropical countries and in sportspersons.
- ✦ Rich vegetarian sources of iron are--dates, gur, (unrefined sugar) bananas, apples, peas, beans, Soya, green vegetables (especially leafy), turmeric, and tamarind. Dairy products are poor sources. Cooking in iron pots increases iron content of food.

Which iron preparations are better?

Haemoglobin containing preparations and those containing ferrous salts are better. There is no particular advantage in any other types. Sustained release preparations may be poorly absorbed and mostly thrown out in stools.

Injectable preparations may be needed in severe anaemia and where a person is totally intolerant to orally administered iron.

What are the side effects of iron therapy?

Iron preparations can cause gastric irritation, constipation and diarrhoea. There are preparations with stool softeners for those patients prone to constipation. Iron can also lead to staining of teeth when given orally, and of the skin when given as an injection. Stools and urine can also turn blackish. (Urine will also look blackish if a person stands for long when he is taking iron preparation). Intra muscular injections can sometimes lead to a severe reaction, therefore a patient should be observed for at least 15 minutes after the first injection. When given intra-venously, it is even more likely to cause a severe reaction; so it is always a good idea to admit a patient to hospital before administering intra venous iron.'

Iodine is an antiseptic, a good steriliser of water, and is also used as a dye injection in various radiological procedures. As iodide, it is present in milk, fish and eggs.

Uses: useful for proper thyroid functioning. Thyroid deficiency can lead to mental retardation, and to prevent this, many governments have made it a policy to iodise common salt. Iodine –deficient water is found along some hilly and & other belts. Those of you suffering from hyper function of thyroid, especially if you eat a balanced diet, may not need to consume iodised salt.

Fibre : It is a very important ' *waste* ' product of food and an essential component of our daily food intake. It can be water soluble or insoluble –

Soluble Fibre: Soluble fibre, holds water to form a gel - like fenugreek, barley, plums, raisins, beans, isapgol, (natural husk) carrots and guar gum etc.

Uses: Consuming enough soluble fibre, gives a feeling of fullness (thereby reducing food intake), softens our stools, and delays absorption of sugar into the blood.

Insoluble fibre: It is found in skins, peels, seeds and husks of fruits and vegetables as also in whole grains.

Uses: It provides bulk to food, softens stools, and traps and throws out fats. Fibre, thus has zero calories, helps in constipation, diarrhoea, weight reduction, diabetes, hyperlipidaemia (increase in bad fats), piles, and even prevents bowel cancer.

So make sure you consume daily five hundred grams of fruits and vegetables, and always eat whole grain cereals so that your body gets enough of this useful substance   unfortunately called a 'waste '.

Fibre thus has zero calories, helps in constipation, diarrhoea, weight reduction, diabetes, hyperlipidaemia (increase in bad fats), piles, and even prevents bowel cancer. Hardly a waste product don't you agree!

Next we talk about a fibre-rich and nutri-rich entity called-sprouts.

Just see what happens when we sprout a seed, whole pulse or legume—

SPROUTS THE NUTRITIONAL WONDER

Caloric content	reduced 15%
Carbohydrate content	reduced 15-30%
Protein content	increased 30%
B complex vitamins	increased 200- 500%
Calcium	increased 34 %
Iron	increased 40%
Potassium	increased 80%
Phosphorous	increased 56%
Vitamin A	increased 285%
Vitamin C	infinite increase
Salt?	

All seeds sesame, groundnuts, melon seeds, flax seeds, sunflower seeds), lentils (whole pulses), and legumes (whole) can be sprouted.

Examples of legumes are peas, dried beans, chick-peas, small black eyed peas etc. But make sure you sprout them at home and use clean water, so that you do not pick up an infection!

Most of the benefits are obtained on consuming raw sprouts.

Chew thoroughly and eat to get almost all your vitamins, minerals, proteins and fibre requirements! You will have seen a question mark after 'salt' - yes, salt content is also increased so reduce your salt intake if you are regularly consuming sprouts.

Spices and Condiments : Not for nothing does spice rhyme with nice. Besides their known flavouring properties, spices also have many medicinal and cosmetic uses. Spices additionally have free radical scavenging properties or anti-oxidant effect and therefore can protect us from many chronic diseases. In fact one clove and one cardamom are said to be enough to provide adequate anti-oxidant protection for a day.

Clove, fenugreek, mustard, turmeric, black pepper, cardamom, red pepper are some of the commonly used spices and condiments, which are very useful.

Uses: They aid in digestion, fight infections, have anti cold properties, reduce body ache, melt body fat, provide fibre, aid in bowel movements, bring down body temperature, strengthen bones and joints, improve appetite and beautify us. Whew! With all these attributes, why under-use them? Use them regularly to fully utilise their attributes and derive maximal benefit.

Variety the Spice of Life

One simple thumb rule to remember---is to eat a variety of foods - fruits, cooked vegetables, salads, sprouts, pulses, grains, dairy products, and spices. The more variety you eat, and the more colours and flavours on your plate, the healthier you are going to be. Balanced diet to me means just that.

So what should you eat? Let me put it very simply since I don't want to burden you with a lot of details-

- ✦ Half a Kg. cooked vegetables - eat all vegetables including bitter ones - include garlic and ginger.

- ✦ Three-five different fruits—spread through the day.

- ✦ Two small bowls of mixed salads-- with minimal dressing and salt.

- ✦ A cup of raw mixed sprouts seeds, flax seeds, sunflower seeds) and legumes can be sprouted.

- ✦ 3 cups of cow's milk with minimal cream, or skimmed cow's milk.

- ✦ 3 cups of buttermilk/low fat curd.

- ✦ Multigrain chapattis, (Indian flat bread), and bread -- made out of whole wheat, soya, millets, and corn.

- ✦ Brown or unpolished rice, alternately, white rice cooked on gas (not in cooker), with the starch drained out.

- ✦ Oats and ragi are high on nutrition and fibre content.

- ✦ All pulses—see that you eat all of them every week.

- ✦ Cooked Legumes and peas—again try to eat as many of them as you can in a week or mix them and cook.

- ✦ 5 teaspoonful cold pressed oil (any cooking oil of your choice.)

- ✦ Half a teaspoonful of salt a day—that's all that's required!

- ✦ For non-vegetarians--Fish and chicken without skin,

white of egg.

✦   Use spices like—

Turmeric—it is an antiseptic, melts fat, beautifies and has anti cancer properties.

Chillies—excellent pain killer, and blood thinner

Cloves and Cardamom—best antioxidants.

Black pepper—burns fats.

Fenugreek—lowers cholesterol and blood sugar.

Cumin seeds—keeps you cool and good digestive.

Cinnamon —reduces blood glucose.

What to avoid as far as possible -

Sugar, sweets, bakery items, fried foods, butter, cheese, ghee(clarified butter), outside snacks, white rice(with undrained starch), refined flour products, salty items--pickles, salted snacks), cream, red meat, egg yolk, refined oils, hydrogenated oils(margarine), re-using oil after deep frying.

Also avoid eating out as far as possible. On an average when you eat in a hotel, you take in four times the calories of home food!!

With this diet, you will stay slim or lose weight if already fat; keep diabetes, blood pressure heart disease and cancer at bay, and have a healthy stomach and bowels. You will also get all the minerals, vitamins, trace elements, carbohydrates, proteins, fats and fiber that you require.

THE VEGETARIAN MANTRA

Vegetarianism is in vogue these days, and it is considered fashionable to proclaim how one has turned green.

Patients need to be convinced with hard facts about the benefits of vegetarianism without being dogmatic, and why it is good to reduce non-vegetarian intake, after the growing years have passed. Let us attempt to do so -

1. Firstly, an animal based diet, is rich in proteins and cholesterol which is further increased in castrated animals. (commonly performed on cattle reared for their meat.)

2. Meat contains no essential nutrients that cannot be obtained from plant sources. By cycling grain through animals, we in fact *lose* 99% carbohydrates and 100% fibre!

3. Chicken feed is routinely laced with hormones and antibiotics to ensure infection-free and healthy stock.

4. Meat centric diets increase our susceptibility to many cancers especially that of colon, breast, cervix, ovaries, prostate and lungs.

5. Human intestines are not designed to digest meat. A carnivore's intestines are relatively short (3 times the length of its body) and smooth inside to facilitate passage of meat. Human intestines however, are 12 times the length of the body, and deeply twisted and puckered from inside and because of lack of fibre in meat, it inches itself through this convoluted passage and before reaching the end, it can become toxic to the body.

6. Meat is rich in iron, but totally lacks vitamin C, which is essential for its absorption (of iron) into the body from the intestines. Lack of vitamin C can also lead to bleeding from gums and skin.

7. Fish absorbs toxic chemicals easily; especially mercury and this may lead to a low sperm count and infertility in men, so try to source your fish from unpolluted waters.

8. Most diet related allergies come from consumption of meat, fish and eggs.

9. Non-vegetarian foods are the sources of many kinds of bacteria, viruses and parasites like tape worm, typhoid bacteria, mad-cow virus etc which may remain active if meat is incompletely cooked.

10. Meat contains approximately 14 times more pesticide than plant food.

11. Most drugs used on animals have not been approved for human use and residues may remain in the meat as there is no proper regulation for drug administration to cattle.

12. Non-vegetarian food by nature is acidic and those who suffer from acidity should cut down its intake.

In short, consuming an animal based diet increases our susceptibility to constipation, obesity, hypertension, heart disease, cancer, acidity, and infections, besides subjecting us to the toxic effects of residual drugs and pesticides. (Fish however is an exception since it is rich in omega –3 fatty acids, which is good for the heart). Reason enough for turning vegetarian-- or at least a fisheatarian?

Ref: - Herald of health May 99 "101 reasons why I'm a vegetarian"

✦ ✦ ✦ ✦

23

Tonics or Toxins

*"A pinch of salt is life saving,
but sea water - is poisonous!"*

In other words- too much of a good thing is not necessarily better.

What do you do when you are feeling debilitated, asthenic, run down? - Reach for your multivitamin, multimineral supplement - right? O.K., take it for a short while and stop. However if you continue to consume them, your *tonic* may actually turn into a *to/in-*

There are certain situations where vitamins or mineral supplements are indicated for a short or long duration. Some of these may be – when our intake of food due to any cause is less or we are suffering from diarrhoea or vomiting OR there is increased demand from our body like - pregnancy, lactation, stress, fevers, post–operative states, old age etc. Besides this, specific supplements will be prescribed by your doctor under conditions of deficiency - like calcium in osteoporosis, (thinning of bones.) and menopausal women, iron in anaemia, folic acid vitamin with epilepsy and cancer drugs, and so on. But regular intake of any supplement, without proper indication can lead to harmful side effects. Newer studies are also revealing that supplementation of anti oxidant vitamins like vitamin C, B – carotene and Selenium may interfere with the action of lipid lowering drugs, and prolonged use of some supplements may increase the incidence of cancer in smokers instead of lowering it.

Now, let us understand how *e/cess* of each supplement can harm us.

B complex vitamins and vitamin C: Since these are water-soluble and any excess is thrown out with urine, they are considered totally safe. In fact you will be surprised at how unsafe they can be.

Excessive intake of B complex vitamins can lead to skin changes, activation of stomach ulcers, precipitate jaundice and diabetes, lead to kidney stone formation, bring about a drop in B.P., cause nerve damage, lead to loss of balance and even fits!

B - Complex injections - those much sought after panaceas for 'weakness' can actually kill, *if there is a reaction.*

Vitamin C - It is called a wonder–drug, and the myths surrounding it are legion - but don't get carried away by any kind of propaganda. Indiscriminate use of this vitamin can impair nerve functions, cause gout, reduce bone growth, lead to kidney stone formation and destroy vitamin B 12 from food. Also, if you are a diabetic, remember – your urine may show false sugar reaction if you are taking vitamin C.

These water-soluble vitamins are relatively safe; but fat-soluble ones get *stored* in the body and act as *slow to/ins.*

Vitamin A: A very useful vitamin in correct doses; but any excess intake even for a short while can lead to problems. In the beginning we can suffer from irritability, vomiting, loss of appetite and headache. Over a longer period of intake, we will have roughening of skin, swollen gums, enlargement of liver and spleen, and even go into fits, or become unconscious!

Vitamin D: Excessive doses can cause fatigue, headache, nausea, diarrhoea, kidney stone formation and even kidney damage.

Vitamin E : In many people, large doses of vitamin E have been given, without apparent serious side effects; but in a few, it can lead to malaise, headache, nausea, fatigue, blurred vision, gastro-intestinal disturbances and even hypertension. In men, it can cause breast enlargement and feminisation. In two classes of people, it should never be used – in *those taking blood-thinning drugs,* in whom it can cause bleeding from various parts of the body, and in infants where life threatening side effects may occur.

Minerals: Minerals like calcium and iron are also commonly taken without actual need. Iron can lead to dyspepsia, constipation, diarrhoea, vomiting and even bleeding from stomach. Iron injections can cause local discolouration of skin, enlargement of lymph nodes, and sometimes lead to a reaction - mild with intramuscular, and severe with intravenous administration. Excessive iron can also get deposited in various organs and damage them over a period of time. There are also certain types of anaemias in which iron should *not* be used—ask your doctor.

Calcium: Calcium is again highly misused. Excessive calcium is deposited in blood vessels and various parts of the body and can lead to hardening of arteries, kidney stone etc. Injectable calcium can cause serious reaction if improperly administered.

Fluoride: A special mention should be made of fluoride, because of the free availability of fluoridated toothpastes. There are certain belts in India & all over the world, where fluoride content of water is very high, so consider the consequences of using fluoridated toothpastes(however minute the fluoride content) by people living in these areas. Too much fluoride can discolour our teeth and stiffen our spine. This is still a controversial subject, with dentists arguing for and against it.

Chromium—doses larger than 200 µg are toxic and can cause difficulty in concentration and fainting.

Copper—more than 10 milligrams can be toxic to nerves and liver.

Magnesium-doses larger than 400 milligrams can cause stomach irritation and diarrhea.

Molybdenum-doses larger than 200 µg can damage the kidneys

Zinc-doses larger than 20milligrams can cause anaemia and copper deficiency

Liquid tonics: Many liquid tonics contain sugar, which should not be taken by diabetics, and worse, some contain alcohol, which can prove addicting especially in children.

So, we have seen how a useful 'tonic' can turn into a harmful 'toxin' when used wrongly. Now you will ask me why excessive intake of vitamins and minerals from food does not harm us. It is important to understand that food contains fibre, which ensures that anything taken in excess is thrown out in the stools –*therefore chances of tolicity are less.*

So, next time you reach for that pill for 'strength', do consult before you pop!

Ref: **-1)** Harrison's principles of medicine, 2) Ann.NY Acad.sci. 82:361 1982, 3), Arch.of internal med140: 1731980, 4) Paediatric76: 625 1985,**5)** Eur.Neurol.14: 340 1976, **6**) N Eng.J Med. 309:445 1983,7) Ann.int. Med.84: 385 1976,**8**) Drugs therapy 26:73 1984 **9**), Dis-A-month 24:1 1983, **10**) Nutr. Rev. 42: 43 1984

✦ ✦ ✦ ✦

24

All about Oil

In this chapter, let us fuel ourselves with all the oily truths we need to know, beginning with how much oil we really need. Actually, after we stop growing, our requirement is only about five-teaspoonfuls a day! That includes everything - from milk fat, curd fat, oil used for cooking, ghee(clarified butter) butter etc. ----. Now imagine how much extra each of us is consuming. There is only one reason more of us do not get our blood vessels fat clogged - it is probably because of the fibre that we consume in large amounts. This fibre traps the excessive oil, and throws it out in the stools.

Which oil should we use?

There is so much misinformation and propaganda about oil, that most people are confused. Well, the best oil is one, which is naturally extracted and does not contain chemical additives or adulterants. Should we use refined oils, and what is this refining? (Our grandmothers did not use refined oil, and if we follow the food and living habits of that generation we would remain healthy.)

Refining - involves removal of free fatty acids, bleaching, and removal of objectionable odours. To achieve this clear, odourless, sanitised state, oil is either subjected to temperatures ranging from 75 – 270 * C, or to addition of chemicals like phosphoric acid and caustic soda! This process destroys natural Beta-carotene and vitamin E (which protects oil from becoming rancid) and leaves toxic residues. So when we buy refined oil, we are paying more, losing vitamins, and may be taking in toxins, which can damage our heart and brain or even cause cancer! I am not saying all refined oils are bad, but how many of them mention date of extraction, toxin and vitamin levels?

If you like oil that looks clear, and the container label shows these particulars (mentioned above), there is no harm in buying it, but a good quality filtered oil may be safer and cheaper-- the best oil being naturally extracted in a cold press.

Storage

Next, let us consider, how oil should be stored. Oil should be stored in good quality steel, glass or earthenware containers and never in plastic or tin ones. Keep your oil in a dark place, away from direct light or heat, to prevent it from disintegrating fast. Do you know that oil should be ideally consumed within a month of extraction? So, buy less oil at a time, and naturally extracted if possible. If you buy packaged oil look out for the following data on the container - date of extraction (and not date of packaging), toxic residue levels and vitamin levels.

Try not to deep-fry your food, at more than 180° C (smoking oil), it can lead to - diarrhoea, vomiting, mental depression, fatty liver etc. To avoid high temperature, use a shallow pan with minimal oil and a low flame. Water in oil is also harmful, and do not re-use oil especially if it contains food residues.

Which oil is best - Obviously, saturated oils like coconut, palm kernel oil, clarified butter, hydrogenated vegetable oil and margarine should not be used for regular cooking.

Among the unsaturated oils - rice bran oil, Soya, fish oil and rapeseed oil– are best for the heart. We do not use fish and rapeseed oil as cooking media. Mustard, til(sesame), soya, rice-bran, and olive oil are good. Corn, groundnut (peanut), and sunflower are also O.K in moderation. Use a combination of these and try to use as many as you can. One or two can be used as cooking media, according to your preference, and the others can be consumed as powders added during cooking. e.g. – mustard, sesame and pea nut powders. A good method is to alternate type of oil used so that you get benefits of different oils.

Don't get carried away by advertisements showing particular oils being used to fry food, and proclaiming such fried food, are *good* for the heart! The main point is not only *which oil* but also *how much* of it, since excessive intake of *any oil* will make us put on weight and there can be nothing worse for the heart than obesity. Consumer activists should question the pertinency of these advertisements.

To summarise, use five teaspoonfuls of oil a day, naturally extracted if possible, use a mixture of oils in various forms, (preferably the oils used by your older generations) choose the right container, store properly, avoid high temperature frying and if you use packaged oil, buy a little at a time and study the label properly before buying!

Ref.: "Judicious use of vegetable oils for a healthy heart, a guide for the family physician. By Dr.Peeyush Jain. Mediquest (Ranbaxy)

✦✦✦✦

25

Dangers of Self Medication

Due to increasing cost of consultations and time constraints, pill popping and self-medication are becoming common. Up to an extent, treating yourselves with the help of chemists, and knowledge culled from the media is O.K., but you must understand the implications of this as by trying to save a little time and money, you may be endangering your health and even life. Some unscrupulous and unqualified chemists may also give you outdated, sub-standard or wrong medicines without your being aware of it.

Vitamin and mineral supplements are the commonest pills to be self-prescribed and the dangers of their long-term over use have been dealt with in the previous chapters.

Next in order of frequency are *painkillers and cold remedies.* These medicines can cause acidity, even severe bleeding from the stomach, fluid retention in body, increase in blood pressure, and even kidney damage, besides which cold remedies can interfere with your concentration powers, precipitate urine retention in a person with enlarged prostate, and cause glaucoma too (increase in fluid pressure in eyes).

Cold & cough remedies with PPA –Many common cold and cough medications, containing PPA, (phenyl propalamine—*it has been banned now)*, can cause bleeding in the brain, which can lead even to sudden death.

Anti diarrhoeals should be taken sparingly since it is not a good idea to 'choke up' diarrhoea and *antispasm drugs* (for stomach colic) should be used with special caution in a case of inflamed appendix or bowel obstruction.

Drugs for hyperacidity

Indiscriminate and prolonged acid suppression can sometimes lead to cancer. Also acid suppression drug called proton pump inhibitor used very commonly can cause magnesium deficiency, leading to irregularity in heart beat, and osteoporosis. It can also lead to vitamin-B-12 and iron deficiency. Omeprazole also interferes with the action of Clopidogrel, a commonly used blood thinning drug.

Drugs for vomiting should always be used with care, since vomiting can be due to jaundice and the patient may go into coma also many of these drugs can cause peculiar distortions of face and body, which may scare the patient or get him wrongly labeled as a psychiatric case.

Electrolyte powders = "energy"? - Many patients equate electrolyte powders with energy. Electrolyte supplementations are needed when there is *loss* due to vomiting, diarrhoea or increased sweating (as in fevers). But patients must understand that their indiscriminate intake can be harmful in patients with blood pressure, kidney damage etc. Electrolytes must therefore be taken only when prescribed by doctors & not randomly for "energy."

Sleeping pills are addicting and should not be taken continuously unless prescribed by your doctor.

Antibiotics taken indiscriminately or in inadequate doses are also dangerous, not only for the person who takes them but for the community too, as resistant strains of bacteria may develop which will not respond to available drugs. So taking antibiotics on your own should definitely be avoided.

If you have *liver, kidney or heart problems,* be very careful about what medicines you take and *diabetics and hypertensives* should not try to treat themselves, as erratic control can lead to complications and don't take cold remedies or anti-amoebic drugs and drive a vehicle, especially if it is also after some cocktails at dinner - you may be heading for trouble.

Dangers of unsupervised and long term use of *steroid ointments and creams* have been discussed in the chapter on Skin.

Pregnancy and children - Although beyond the scope of this book, I am highlighting the misuse of drugs in pregnancy and children, as this is very important. In the first three months of pregnancy, as far as possible, no medication should be taken including vitamins, as the foetus is in the stage of development and congenital deformities can occur (except folic acid vitamin which prevents deformities). Caution has to be exercised during lactation (breast feeding) also, since the drugs taken by the mother may affect the child. As for children, always remember the dictum "Child is not a compressed adult". Children should not take aspirin containing medications, tetracycline and quinolone group of drugs etc. and it is important to give medicines only according to body weight of the child.

Now that you are aware of the dangers of self-prescribed medications, exercise caution next time you take drugs on your own for common ailments. It will be safer to consult your doctor and keep a set of common drugs, which can be used after telephonically consulting her/ him regarding their safety and side effects.

Dangers of admission to hospital

There are many patients who like to get admitted to hospital for fluid adminstration, ("saline and glucose") thinking it will give them strength, and others want to be admitted for routine fevers and minor ailments. It is important to understand that admission in hospital will increase their chances of acquiring *Nosocomial* (hospital) infections from other patients, which may be very difficult to cure; hence admissions should be encouraged only where really needed.

26

Some Useful Discomforts

That discomforts can be useful, sounds like a paradox, but some of our complaints are like bitter foods, difficult to tolerate, but as any grandmother worth her age will corroborate, good for us.

Pain, fever, a flowing nose, cough, swelling and sweating are some of the weapons in the body's armory, which defend us from external aliens like infections, toxins and allergens, so are useful to us.

Pain

Consider pain for example, 50% of patients coming to doctors, present with this complaint and if it weren't for it, we would not come to know that we were suffering from a heart attack, kidney stone or acute appendicitis, would we?

Leprosy patients have their nerves destroyed by their illness, and because of consequent loss of pain sensation, do not realise that they are being gnawed by rats or burnt by fire, thus losing parts of their fingers or toes. When pain is severe, it should definitely be alleviated, but in chronic cases, it is important to use methods to alter *perception* to pain rather than use long-term medications with their potential side effects.

Next let us consider fever-

Fever

Every time I see a case of fever, I get chills down *my* spine, because fever is such an unpredictable condition, and the causes are so many that occasionally, even in the most experienced hands, things can go awry. This is best illustrated by the following joke –

A patient came to a doctor with fever and cold and was given some medicines to bring it down. After two days, he was back with the complaint that the fever was continuing, so an antibiotic was started. Two days later, he went back to the doctor, now extremely peeved, and demanded, "doctor, can this fever be controlled?" "Yes", says the doctor "go home, take a cold shower (it was winter!) And with a wet body, stand in front of an open window"

"But" says the patient, "I will get pneumonia"! "Right", replies the doctor, "that's the idea, *Pneumonia,* I can treat!"

Most patients are surprised that it sometimes takes many days to bring a fever under control and are ready to brand doctors as incompetent because of this. They need to understand that there are hundreds of causes of fever, and typical presentations are not seen nowadays. Gone are the days when a patient had classical symptoms of tuberculosis, typhoid or malaria. Because of rampant misuse of antibiotics, no fever conforms to its textbook picture.

Another thing patients need to be made aware of is that *antibiotic* is not a single umbrella drug which can cure every fever. Just as there are numerous types and causes of fever, there are many antibiotics used to treat them, and no single antibiotic can cure all fevers. Doctors have to consider many factors before choosing an antibiotic, such as whether the patient has any disease or problem in which a particular antibiotic should not be used, any previous history of drug allergy etc. Therefore, even if a certain antibiotic is indicated in a problem, we may not be able to use it because of contra indications. So every time do not expect sure shot results.

While on this topic, let me caution you against taking self-prescribed antibiotics especially in inadequate doses or for a shorter period than prescribed. It can create dangerous resistance which is harmful not only to you, but to the community at large.

Now what are the causes of fever?

1.   The most common cause is due to infections, which may be bacterial, viral, fungal, protozoal etc.

2.   Sometimes it is *drug* induced,(as a reaction to some drug which you are taking)

3.   It may be due to acute inflammation or swelling, due to any cause

4.   Due to thrombotic (blocks in blood vessels) conditions

5.   Certain cancers present with fever

6.   Certain diseases like gout, hyper- active thyroid etc

7.   Due to heat stroke

8.   Due to foreign substance in body – the body reacts with fever in order to expel the foreign substance.

9.   Normal' fever – there are some patients, in whom a slight rise of body temperature is always present, but no cause is found and reassurance is the only treatment required.

10.   Lastly, fever can be self-induced. This can be done by various ingenious methods, which I would rather not elaborate on!

This is normally resorted to by people who want to bunk their duties or more commonly in psychiatric cases.

Benefits of fever:

It is extremely important to understand that *fever is good for us.* It is a state of heightened reaction by the body, in order to fight an infection or abnormal state, so obviously it is NOT a good idea to suppress it.

When and how to treat it

Since fever is beneficial to us, any mild increase in temperature should be left alone since we may be interfering with the body's ability to deal with a more severe infection at a later date.

Injections to suppress fever should only be given in the following conditions:

a.   Heat stroke

b.   In a person prone to febrile (fever induced) fits and

c.   When fever is so high that it may damage the brain and other vital organs (beyond 105*F.)

In most other cases, *using injections to bring down fever* is like using a sword to kill a mosquito, not only useless, but also potentially harmful. Firstly, there may be a severe reaction due to the injection, secondly we are interfering with the body's mechanism of fighting an infection; thirdly the patient may get a false sense of well-being and over-exert only to come down with a severe relapse, and lastly, the typical pattern of a fever may be lost, making diagnosis difficult without investigations.

Swelling

Next we deal with swelling. In an attempt to throw out a foreign body or infection, the body pours out cells and fluids into the affected part trying to scavenge unwanted substances, and drain them away. Since this is a healing reaction, we must not suppress this swelling totally and take only mild anti-inflammatory drugs, and rest the part, while allowing the body to do its job.

A flowing nose and cough

These are again good for us because they are methods of dealing with upper respiratory infections or allergens. They should be treated only

a. If they last beyond 15 days

b. There is a dry hacking cough with breathing difficulty

c. Or it is accompanied by fever.

Another thing to understand is that cough syrups are of various kinds and it is important to use the correct type. For example, using a cough suppressant for a productive cough may 'choke' it up and lead to fever.

Sweating

Lastly let us deal with the complaint of sweating. In these days of appearing well groomed, no one wants to appear sweaty, but sweating not only lowers our body temperature (by losing heat), it throws out toxins, burns fat, and is a natural moisturizer for the skin, so don't be embarrassed at 'sweating it out!'

In conclusion, let us again remember that all these so called discomforts are good for us because they are outward manifestations of the body's attempt to deal with foreign substances and they tell us that all is well with our defense system. So, next time we suffer from an illness, let us thank these *allies*, who we have so far regarded as *enemies*, for helping our body to heal itself, and use only mild supportive measures but never ham-handed ones to suppress them. But sometimes as with all security forces, the body does tend to over-react and here, 'masterly inactivity' should immediately give way to 'judicious intervention' as and when required. It is important therefore to remain under medical supervision.

++++

27

Rights of Patients and Doctors

"Only the dutiful, deserve their rights."

If patients know and exercise their rights judiciously, it will prevent unpleasant situations from taking place inadvertently. A doctor – patient relationship has to be based on faith and trust. You must understand that the human body is not a machine and no two people are alike. Doctors base their judgment of a disease and subsequent management, on previous experience, evidence based studies and textbook knowledge. Occasionally, a patient may not respond in a textbook manner, and things may go wrong. If he is an enlightened person, he will discuss with the doctor all the merits and demerits of different treatment modalities, and there will be no controversy later, regarding any results of therapy.

So what are your rights?

1. First and most important is a right to a prescription. Every doctor is obliged to give you a prescription and if they don't, insist on it. The prescription should have the doctor's name, address, phone number and registration number, name of patient, date, diagnoses, complaints,

examination-findings, investigations advised and treatment given. Also, don't accept any unlabelled drugs; they may be from some sub-standard manufacturers.

Similarly when admitted to any hospital or nursing home, make sure you collect your discharge card. Discharge card should state your name, address, age, doctor's name, hospital's name and address, and date of admission and discharge, proper history, examination-findings, investigations done, line of management, final prescription, diagnoses and doctor's signature. This is a very important document and especially if you are covered under mediclaim, comes in very useful, so make sure all entries are complete. In history, especially duration of complaints is important for mediclaim insurance – so make sure it is entered in the discharge card.

2. **Your second right is right to information**. - At any time you have a right to request the doctor for any part of your record kept with him or at a hospital.

3. **Right of knowledge of treatment** - you have a right to know about the medications being given to you and to find out if any possible precautions need to be observed while taking these medicines.

4. **Right of knowledge of Investigation** - You should understand why any investigation is being advised and what it will cost before going in for the test.

5. **Right of choice of referral doctor or hospital -**.

    Doctors will usually refer you to a place where you will get good service, but if you have any individual preferences don't hesitate to say so.

6. **Right to request a second opinion** if you feel it is

required.

7. **Right to privacy** - You have a right to be examined with dignity and in privacy.

8. **Right of full knowledge of any surgery or procedure** before giving consent.

9. **Right of knowledge of being included in any research process.**

10. **Right to avail of treatment in case of an emergency**. No doctor or hospital can refuse an emergency case if no other alternative is available. It is against their ethics.

Remember, doctors are professionals and have to maintain their reputation – hence, they will not commit mistakes on purpose. Also don't waste their time with frivolous complaints and always keep your queries brief and to the point.

Finally choose your doctor with care, avoiding quacks, semi-wise, semi-fools, and the 'cure-it-all', 'know-it-all' types, & those who give guarantees of cure; there is no guarantee in medicine and you could be putting your life in danger, besides wasting a lot of money and time.

Patients' responsibilities

You also have some responsibilities—

1. Responsibility to understand and exercise your rights judiciously.

2. Responsibility of understanding everything about a procedure or operation before giving consent.

3. Responsibility of accepting consequences of any management after giving consent.

4. Responsibility of following doctor's advice and instructions meticulously.

5.   Responsibility of providing full information to doctor regarding health and any other medication being taken from any other doctor for any purpose.

Doctors' rights

It is important for patients to understand that doctors also have rights.

1.   Right to choose place and time and type of practice.

2.   Right to fix fees.

3.   Right to choose patients and to refuse anyone except in an emergency.

Doctor can refuse to see a patient

1.   If (s) he is unwell.

2.   Has social function, illness or bereavement in family.

3.   Patient does not belong to his specialty or beyond his/her capacity.

4.   Doctor has consumed alcohol or a sedative.

5.   If the doctor's relationship with the patient is strained.

6.   When the patient has not followed instructions in the past.

7.   If the patient refuses to give written consent for any management.

8.   If the patient demands a specific line of treatment which the doctor thinks is inappropriate.

If the patient is new, the doctor can refuse to see him citing security reasons, especially at night.

✦✦✦✦

28

Some Investigative
and
Surgical Techniques explained

When in doubt---investigate, and when sure   operate

The older we grow, the more investigative procedures we need to undergo and most of these relate to the field of Radiology. It is important to understand exactly what these procedures are, their uses, and limitations.

1. **X – ray – or Roentgenography** - Here X–rays emitted from a machine, penetrate the human body and are exposed onto a film kept on the other side. This is then processed like a photographic film, and a radiograph is obtained. X-ray basically helps us in diagnosing conditions of our skeletal system and to some extent that of soft tissues like chest.

2. **Contrast Radiography** – Here either a dye or barium is injected or drunk, and a series of x-rays taken, to study gastro intestinal tract, kidneys, parts of the vascular system etc. *Angiography* is a form of contrast radiography where the degree of block in the heart and other blood vessels can be assessed.

3. **C T SCAN -** or Computed axial topography, fetched a

Nobel Prize for its inventors. With an ordinary X-ray, only one axis view of a part could be obtained. Here a high energy X-ray beam is passed through the body, and a powerful computer system is used to record images in multiple axes, analyse and even give an opinion. This is very useful for diagnosis of conditions of brain (tumour, bleeding), abdomen and chest. High resolution chest C T and spiral and multi splice C T are newer additions. CT angiography can also be performed.

4. **M R I or magnetic resonance imaging,** entails using a powerful magnet, radio frequency transmitters and special coils to obtain an image. It is safer and more accurate than C T scan and very useful for diagnosing diseases of brain, spine and joints.

    MR angiography (to study blood vessels) and *M R spectroscopy* (to study brain function) are also available .

5. **Interventional radiography** - Here the radiologist participates in both diagnosis and treatment of the patient like in treating narrowed arteries or blocks, removal of kidney and gall stones, treating tumours locally with medication through tubes, closing bleeding blood vessels, again through tubes (catheters) etc.

6. **Ultra sonography-**

    Here high frequency sound waves are generated, which penetrate the human body. The returning echoes are picked up as images by a computerised machine and displayed on a monitor. Ultrasound is very useful for diagnosis of problems of abdomen, pelvis, pregnant ladies, heart and blood vessels. Ultra sound can also be used to treat a frozen shoulder (painful and fixed shoulder) and break kidney and gall stones without surgery.

It is also called *echocardiography* (study of heart with ultrasound) or *colour Doppler* (another word for ultrasound) of heart or blood vessels, where colour is added to appreciate any decrease / increase in flow or turbulence due to obstructions.

7. **E C G** - or electro cardiogram is a test where electrodes are placed on various parts of the body and the electrical activity of the heart is picked up from these points in the form of a graph. ECG tells us not only about the heart but also about numerous diseases in the body like thyroid problems, electrolyte imbalance etc.

8. **E M G** - or electro-myogram is study of the electrical activity of muscles to diagnose various diseases called myopathies or to judge the condition of muscles in neurological diseases.

9. **Nerve conduction studies** to study conditions of various nerves and to detect neuropathy.

10. **E E G** – (Electro encephalogram) to study electrical activity in brain, for diagnosing various types of epilepsy and sleep disorders. It can also be used to certify death. A flat EEG indicates no electrical activity in brain. Normally brain death follows when heart stops and cannot be revived within eight minutes, leading to oxygen deficiency to brain cells and their death, revealed by a flat EEG.

11. **Electro physiology studies** – to detect and to type (classify) various defects in electrical activity of heart and also peripheral nerves.

12. **Bone densimetry-** Density of bone reduces with age, leading to its thinning called *osteoporosis* (porous bones). Sonography or X – ray can be used to measure thickness of bones and evaluate those patients in need of intensive treatment and also help in assessing results of therapy.

13. **Nuclear medicine** - Certain radioactive isotopes are administered to the patient, and various scans done, for example radioactive iodine for thyroid (used both for diagnosis and treatment of thyroid disease).

Thallium scans for heart - for diagnosis of ischaemia (less blood supply) or infarct (dead tissue). Other common scans are – lung, bone, kidneys, liver, intestines (Technetium scan)

1. Positron emission tomography- (PET)

This is a nuclear medicine imaging technique that produces a three-dimensional image or picture of functional processes in the body. Pairs of gamma rays are emitted indirectly by a positron-emitting radionuclide (tracer), which is introduced into the body on a biologically active molecule. The system then detects these gamma rays and three-dimensional images of tracer concentration within the body are then constructed by computer analysis using a CT X-ray scan performed on the patient during the same session, in the same machine

It is used heavily in clinical oncology (medical imaging of tumors and the search for cancer spread), and for clinical diagnosis of certain diffuse brain diseases such as those causing various types of dementias. PET is also an important research tool to map normal human brain and heart function.

PET is also used in pre-clinical studies using animals, where it allows repeated investigations into the same subjects. This is particularly valuable in cancer research,

Remember most of these investigative techniques are relatively new and M R I or sonography as of today are considered safer than X-ray based tests, but we still do not know about their long-term safety, hence it is important to understand from your doctor implications of each test before going in for them, and do them only if they are essential.

✦✦✦✦

30

Medical Check-up After Forty

An ounce of prevention is worth a pound of cure

Once in two years, and preferably every year, it is advisable to go in for a full medical check-up. There are various centers offering schemes for this, but a lot of unnecessary tests are being done. It is better to go to your physician, have a full examination and, let her/him decide what needs to be done.

As a general rule, following tests may be done (extra ones will be advised, as per need)

WOMEN ABOVE FORTY:

1. **Haemogram** – which tells us many things like level of haemoglobin, whether the other blood cells are less or more (infection, leukaemia, bone marrow suppression etc.) - any parasites like malaria and filaria, any abnormality in shape of cells etc.

2. **E S R** - This is the rate at which the red cells settle down in a tube. If there is inflammation in the body, certain sticky proteins increase in the blood, and so the cells settle faster. It helps us especially to chart progress or regression of inflammation in the body.

3. **Blood Glucose** – fasting and after meals, to detect diabetes

4. **Routine urine examination** -

   Examination of urine will tell us if we have diabetes (sugar in urine), any Kidney damage (albumin, certain cells), infection (increase in pus cells) Bleeding (increase in red blood cell) stone formation (increase in crystals), jaundice (increase in bile products) and many other things.

5. **Lipid Profile** - The pattern of fats in our blood --- Fats have been discussed in 'Prevention and management of heart disease' in detail.

6. **Serum Uric Acid** - increase in serum uric acid can lead to gout, joint problems and kidney damage.

7. **Serum Calcium** - an important investigation, as osteoporosis (bone softening) is common after menopause and we need to know how much calcium to substitute. It is also a marker of other diseases.

8. **E C G** - to know the condition of our heart.

1. **A thorough eye examination** – especially in diabetes and hypertensives to detect retinal problems, and in all to detect cataract and glaucoma.

10. **Mammography** every two years -

    This is a special X–ray for detection of breast cancer

11. **Routine Gynaecological examination** & pap smear to detect any cancer. (Covered in chapter on menopause)

12 **Stool** for microscopic blood - to detect cancer of colon (large intestines) & any infection or infestation (with worms)

13. **Abdomino pelvic sonography** - may be done once in two years to detect small tumour, kidney or gall stone.

All these tests need not be done every year. Your doctor will decide what should be done and also add some new ones as required.

I have purposely not included X–ray chest. X-ray should be conducted only if necessary. *Remember each time you go in for an X–ray, you are adding to your radiation e/posure, and increasing your chances of getting cancer.*

MEN ABOVE FORTY:
1. Haemogram.
2. ESR.
3. Blood Glucose.
4. Lipid Profile.
5. Liver function tests.
6. Urine.
7. Stool.
8. PSA (Prostate specific antigen) if prostate is enlarged.
9. Eye check – up.
10. Abdomino pelvic testicular sonography — especially for testes, liver, prostate and urinary stones.
11. Serum Uric acid.
12. ECG
13. X – ray chest if smoker .

Others - tailored accordingly to individual requirement.

Remember, main examination should be a *thorough* physical examination by your doctor. The record kept by him/her will also reveal any changes in the reports as compared to previous years, which can prove very useful.

✦✦✦✦

31

Few First Aid Hints

"A stitch in time-----can save a life."

1. Washing with running tap water is the best first aid for burns, but remember to ensure that the water pressure is not too high. Remember, also that   bandaging a burn tightly, can prove to be dangerous. Never cover a burn with a greasy substance like butter. It will seal it off and retain all the heat inside. Remove all tight clothing, which may stick to the body but only if it comes off easily. Place strips of clean cloth over the burnt parts.

2. In case of bleeding, apply pressure above the bleed or tie a tourniquet (Bandage). For nosebleed, pinch nostrils, apply ice to forehead and raise head.

3. If a patient *faints*, make him smell something strong, slap him hard once and raise his feet. If conscious, he can be made to sit with his head bent between his knees.

4. If a patient chokes on a foreign body, apply sudden upward pressure with fist of one hand on upper stomach (below breast bone), while supporting back with the other hand. If you are alone and choke, press your chest against a railing or chair to try to dislodge the foreign body.

5. Steaming him in a bathroom will help a choked asthmatic patient. He should also be made to sit on the floor with his head resting on his folded arms (shown in chapter on asthma)

6. If a patient has a heart attack, give a tablet of Aspirin (300 milligrams) if he is conscious. Then feel the pulse in the neck (as shown in the picture below), -if no pulse is felt, give a firm thump to the middle of the chest with closed fist, and then start cardiopulmonary resuscitation (as shown in the picture) till help arrives.

    Chest pain: All chest pains need not be of cardiac (heart) origin. Chest pain can be due to acidity (the commonest cause), muscle pain, and bony cage pain or due to lungs and pleura (cover of the lungs). It may even be due to spondylites (from neck). Sometimes it may be difficult to differentiate, but the first thing to do is to take fast acting and effective antacids. If pain is not relieved, take an aspirin. If there is pain on pressing the chest, it is more likely to be a muscular or bony pain, and if it is a retrosternal (behind breast bone) burn, more likely to be due to hyperacidity, especially if it increases on lying down. Cardiac pain is normally very severe, feels akin to a vice like grip, is accompanied by sweating, and normally radiates to the left upper limb. But sometimes even a doctor may not be able to differentiate the various pains without an electrocardiogram and other investigations. If antacids and a painkiller do not work or if the patient looks serious, call an ambulance or rush the patient to hospital on your own!

7. Take all bites seriously, and always report to your doctor. Snake bites - apply bandage above bite, suck out wound, wash thoroughly with water and rush to hospital within half an hour. Scorpion bites – act same as snake bite.

Medicine chest and first aid box

Every home should have a medicine chest, which should be regularly replenished. A few essential medicines are:

1. Paracetamol tablets (crocin, metacin) for fever

2. Aspirin for heart attack. (The single most useful first line of treatment when a patient is suspected of having an attack). It can be used for headache also but with an antacid.

3. An anti allergic.

4. Anti spasmodic for stomach colic

5. A good antacid – the commonest problem after forty is acidity. Discuss with your doctor, which antacids are more effective and act rapidly especially during sleep– it may avoid many sleepless nights for you (and your doctor!)

6. First aid box can contain cotton, bandage, band-aid, antiseptic solution, antibiotic cream, scissors and tweezers.

7. It should also contain emergency numbers of hospitals, doctors and ambulances. In fact in a real emergency don't call your doctor, call an ambulance or rush the patient to the hospital on your own. A single doctor can do very little by himself in an emergency and precious time may be wasted.

Consult your doctor while equipping your first aid box; and don't forget to inform any new doctor about previous allergies especially to drugs.

Finally, at least one member of the family should be trained in first aid. Lives can be saved if proper first aid is given at the site of an emergency.

CASE STUDIES:

Mr. K had a bout of chest pain and vomiting. A doctor was called in who had no E C G machine, no emergency equipment and little ability to handle an emergency. Mr. K died.

Mrs. G had severe chest pain. The doctor rushed with an E C G machine and emergency bag. Single handedly doing ECG, giving emergency medication, and administering cardio pulmonary resuscitation was impossible and Mrs. G also died.

Mr. S had a severe chest pain. The doctor told him to take an aspirin on phone and on reaching the home of the patient, rushed him to an ICCU without bothering about any home management. Mr. S, although he had a very severe heart attack, was saved and is alive.

These three cases illustrate that in a real emergency, time should not be wasted and the patient should be rushed to the hospital by any means. Never mind if it is a false alarm. One life saved is equal to ten false alarms. A single doctor can really do very little with a serious patient. It requires a trained team to handle a situation like this, so a well-equipped ambulance will prove more useful hence in a confirmed emergency call an ambulance, and not your doctor.

CARDIO – PULMONARY- RESCUSCITATION (CPR)

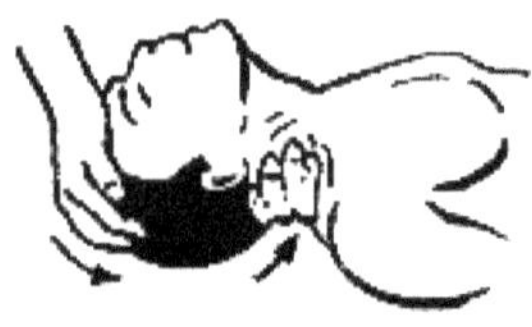

Extend neck, open mouth and look for any foreign objects and remove if easily possible

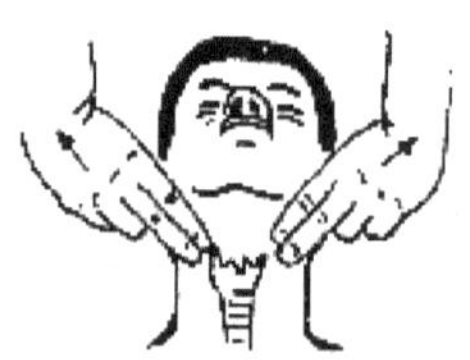

Look for pulse as shown

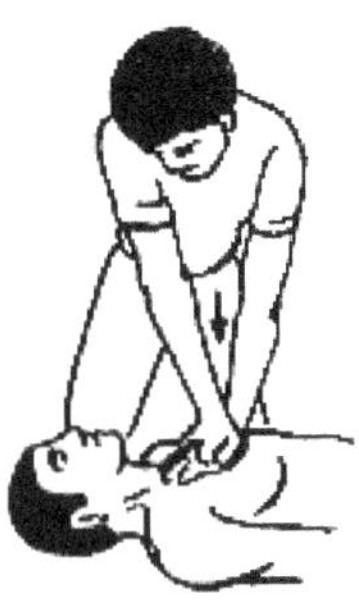
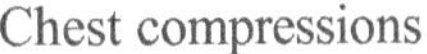
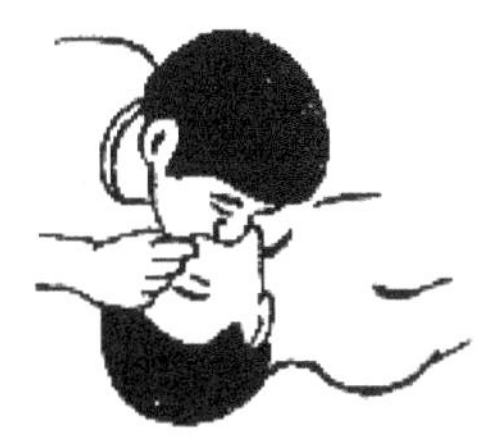

Chest compressions   Mouth – to mouth breathing

CADIO PULMONARY RESCUSCITATION (Pictures above)

As per new American heart association guidelines--2010

CPR - If patient can be moved, shift him from the bed to a firm surface preferably the floor. Give a thump on the breastbone once. Now feel for the pulse in the neck. If no pulse is felt proceed further—remember, chest compressions are of paramount importance and should be started as soon as possible because there is a condition called 'ventricular fibrillation' that can be corrected by early cardiac massage -

CARDIAC MASSAGE-

- Place palm of one hand on lower part of breast bone
- Place heel of the other hand on the first one
- Now keeping the hands straightened, press downwards about 5 centimeters & release abruptly.
- Wait for full recoil of chest before next compression.
- Continue this 100 times a minute.

AIRWAYS

A second operator if available can clear dentures and other foreign objects from mouth before starting artificial respiration. If there is only one operator, he should clear airways only after a few initial chest compressions.

MOUTH-TO-MOUTH BREATHING- After 6-8 seconds of chest compressions, the operator should place his mouth on that of the patient after taking a deep and full breath. Now keeping the patient's nostrils pinched, he should breathe in fully into the latter's mouth. Cardiac massage and mouth-to-mouth breathing (ideal 8-10 per minute) can be performed by two operators for better results, and should be continued till the patient is shifted to hospital or he recovers.

Heart attack when alone

If you are alone and have a heart attack don't panic. Take an aspirin, try to call for help and remember if your heart almost stops beating you have only 10 seconds to revive it. Here's what you can do. Start taking a deep breath and follow it by a deep cough (like we do when we want to remove phlegm from deep inside our chest). Repeat deep breathing followed by coughing every two seconds till help arrives. Deep breaths will push in more oxygen into the lungs and the coughing will stimulate heart and increase circulation of blood. So you see it is like a self administered CPR.

33

The Aging Body

All living things are genetically programmed to start aging when reproductive life ends.

Aging results from cumulative spontaneous mutations (drastic changes) in genes and from errors in the synthesis of proteins critical to the synthesis of genetic material.

The longer we live, the hardier we are. Average life expectancy is now 17 years at age 65, 11 years at age 75, 6 years at age 85, 4 years at age 90, and 2 years at age 100.

The aged differ from the young in several ways.

They normally do not present with the typical presentations of disease. For example a diabetic has a rapid pulse, dizziness and sweating when his blood sugar goes down, but these warning symptoms are absent in the old. Similar is the case with a patient suffering from hyper function of thyroid glands. Even when they have an infection, they do not present with high fever, and so the infection may remain undetected.

Older persons also develop complications of diseases early, like retention of urine in mild prostatic enlargement, diabetic coma when blood sugar is too low or too high, etc.

Drugs are likely to produce side effects at lower doses. For example, some cough and cold remedies and drugs used for depression, can lead to glaucoma or urinary retention (especially in males with mild prostate enlargement), diuretics may lead to urinary incontinence, anti allergic drugs can produce mental confusion.

The only factor that has proven benefits in delaying aging is caloric restriction. The benefit of restricting caloric intake by 30 to 40% has been seen in multiple species, from single-cell organisms to mice. It not only increases average life expectancy but also delays the onset of age-related diseases. Type of food intake does not seem to matter so much like reduction in fats, sugar or salt, as does the reduction in *total* calorie intake. Again, vitamin or antioxidant supplements do not matter to a significant degree as far as increasing life span goes.

However there are some *advantages* of aging! In people who suffer from allergies and vascular headaches (migraines), the frequency and severity actually *reduces.*

And since nerve endings in the skin reduce, sensitivity to pain also reduces!

Now let us see how each part of the body is affected----

Cells

Aging cells are programmed by the body to die by committing a kind of suicide that is called 'apoptosis'. Old cells die because they cannot divide anymore. The length of 'telomeres' on genes decides the life of a cell. With repeated cell division, telomeres shorten and the cell can no longer divide resulting in its death.

Organs

Function of organs becomes less efficient when we age. Partly this is due to reduction in the number of functioning cells. It can also be due to other effects of aging—for example cataract reduces vision, and hardening of arteries reduces function of heart, brain and kidneys. Most body functions start declining slowly as we age. But the effects may not be immediately discernible, because each organ is equipped with a huge number of spare cells and they continue to replace dead cells.

But with a significant decline in cells, older people will find they are less able to cope with excessive work load, extremes of temperature etc.

Brain and Nervous System

We are born with about a trillion nerve cells called neurons and about 3 times the number of supporting or 'glial cells'. We utilise just a small percentage of these cells, so even if we lose a lot of brain cells when we age, it does not matter unless there is a rapid loss of cells (as seen in Alzheimer's disease). Secondly, new connections form between cells to compensate loss of cells from an area. And thirdly there is evidence now that new cells also continue to form even in old age.

Besides decline in number of cells, there is also reduction in the chemicals called neurotransmitters that send and receive messages in the nervous system.

Blood flow to the brain also reduces due to hardening of arteries.

Because of all these changes there is gradual reduction in short term memory, effective speech, and ability to learn and recall new things.

There is also reduction in conduction of messages at the level of spinal and peripheral nerves leading to a slight reduction in sensations.

Heart and blood vessels

We know that our arteries harden as we age. Because of this they lose their elasticity and cannot expand easily, resulting in rise in pressure inside their lumen which we call blood pressure. Because they harden, they also become narrow, and so less blood reaches different parts of the body, especially the heart kidneys and brain—leading to decline in the functions of these organs. But those who exercise regularly will have less arterial hardening even in their old age and thus will retain functions of all their organs.

Reproductive system

Changes are more drastic and sudden in women when they undergo menopause leading to a sudden decline in the levels of oestrogen hormone, leading to shrinking of ovaries and uterus, loss of breast shape, increase in blood pressure, intolerance to heat, and dryness of vagina.

In men the changes are more gradual--- with increasing age there is reduction in libido and impotence.

Lungs

As we age, a number of air sacs in our lungs get clogged with dirt and smoke—obviously more in smokers. The breathing passages and cells also become less elastic. This will hamper strenuous physical activity especially at high altitudes. Cough reflex also becomes weaker so that we are less able to throw out infecting organisms and pollutants, resulting in repeated lung infections. Additionally, muscles of the chest that aid in respiration also become weaker in an older person, adding to the problem.

Bones, Muscles and Joints

If there is one system that bothers an older person the most, it is the skeletal system.

The most dramatic change is in the density of bones especially in females due to reduction in oestrogen levels after menopause. This leads to brittle bones and fractures. Exposure to sunlight, exercise, a good diet, and supplementation with calcium and vitamin D will reduce this problem.

Spinal vertebrae become thinner and the cushion between them also wares off leading to spondylitic changes, fractures, and also shortening of overall height.

Cartilage that lines joints gets frayed, ligaments (that bind the joints) and tendons (that join muscles to bone), become less elastic leading to stiffness, loss of flexibility and arthritis.

Muscle mass steadily declines after the age of thirty especially in those who are sedentary by nature or occupation. This is because of lowering of levels of growth hormone (in both sexes) and testosterone (in males). Loss of muscle mass is less in those who continue with physical exercise. On the other hand, it is rapid in the bed-ridden.

Body fat

If there is a decline in muscle mass, there is doubling of body fat as we age. Distribution of body fat also matters. Fat accumulation around the organs inside the abdomen (visceral fat) is the worst and leads to diabetes and blood pressure. This is because fat accumulation here, interferes with the action of insulin. Insulin levels increase in the blood leading to rise in blood pressure. Since the insulin cannot act, there is a condition called 'insulin resistance' leading to inability of the cells to take in sugar. Thus accumulation of sugar in blood leads to diabetes. Again this problem is less in those who exercise regularly and keep their diets under control.

Digestive system

The 'sphincter' that closes the oesophagus and prevents

regurgitation of food back into the throat becomes lax resulting in heart burn, an irritant cough and eructations. Stomach also empties more slowly and there is reduction in digestive enzymes leading to 'gas' and bloating. The intestines also move slowly resulting in constipation. Action of liver also becomes sluggish so it is not able to release glucose quickly in an emergency in a diabetic resulting in hypoglycaemia (low blood sugar) leading to fainting and even unconsciousness. Drugs and toxins are also not destroyed fast enough by the liver leading to toxicity.

Eyes

We all know that around the age of forty, the lens starts becoming opaque due to cataract leading to reduction in near vision. With aging, the pupils also adjust less efficiently to light—so there maybe a need for brighter lighting Some people also experience the reverse—that is a feeling of 'glare' or intolerance to bright light.. Incidence of glaucoma (increased fluid pressure in eyes) also goes up. There is reduction in the secretion of lubricating fluid from the glands, resulting in dryness. 'Floating' particles are also perceived by many people. These are harmless unless they are too many in number resulting in interference with vision. Eyes may also lose their brightness and appear sunken due to loss of facial fat.

Ears

Hearing loss is something that almost all old people suffer from to a greater or lesser degree. In many of them it is due to longstanding exposure to loud noise, in only a few it is due to old age itself. Old people find it difficult to hear high pitched sounds, and in fact it maybe easier to communicate with them by speaking slowly and enunciating each word clearly, rather than speaking loudly and fast.

Mouth

Like the eyes, mouth also tends to get dry due to reduced salivation. Taste sensitivity also goes down especially for salt and sweet. Gums also recede, leading to exposure of roots of teeth to infections.

Nose

Sense of smell reduces, which also affects taste of food since taste also depends upon flavour or aroma of food. Drying up of the nose also interferes with the ability to fight infections.

Skin

Skin becomes thin and due to loss of elasticity it shows fine wrinkles. This is because of reduction in collagen content of skin. Due to loss of fat, the rounded look also goes away and sensitivity to cold goes up. Blood flow to skin is reduced, leading to delay in wound healing. Old people are less likely to go out in the sun and the vitamin D level in their skin also reduces leading to deficiency of this vitamin and weak bones.

Kidneys and urinary system

Blood supply to the kidneys reduces, leading to less efficient toxic elimination. Muscles of urinary bladder become weak and it finds it difficult to retain urine for long. The external sphincter (that is under voluntary control) becomes lax and urine may flow out without control. In men the prostate gland enlarges leading to blockage in the urinary passage leading to difficulty in passing urine that may require surgery.

Hormonal changes

We know that oestrogen levels reduce drastically during menopause in females and there is a gradual reduction in testosterone levels in males. Growth hormone also reduces leading to reduction in muscle mass, and insulin levels reduce, increasing chances of diabetes. Levels of aldosterone, a water retaining hormone also reduce, leading to dryness and even dehydration.

Anaemia

Due to a slight reduction in production of blood cells and improper diet, anaemia is more common in the old.

Reduced immunity

Immune cells also reduce leading to repeated attacks of infections and even cancer.

FALLS

Falls are a major problem for elderly people.

Causes of Falls With age, balance becomes impaired, muscles and bones become weak, reaction time and reflexes weaken, and vision deteriorates, leading to falls. Falls may also be due to medications or vertigo caused by middle ear infection. Sometimes an ischaemic attack in the brain or a low blood sugar can also cause a person to fall. A defective and uneven floor or a hole in the road or an unexpected obstruction can result in a fall. Alcohol consumption impairs reflexes and can result in a fall. Falls can occur after meals due to fall in blood pressure.

Complications of falls

Falls can result in fractures that can immobilize a person for many months leading to further degenerative changes. They can lead to bleeding inside the brain, (sub dural haematoma). This should be especially looked for if the patient has a severe headache or is confused within a week of a fall.

Prevention

Falls can be prevented by observing the following precautions -

At home

Ensure adequate lighting

Railing in stairs and in the bathroom

Rough non-slippery floors

Avoid self-medication

Detect and treat osteoporosis

Avoid clutter

Have a regular check up

Wear good glasses

Avoid hurried movements

Avoid climbing on unwieldy stools, ladders and furniture

Avoid clothes that make you trip

Outside the home

Carry a walking stick

Venture out in daylight only

Avoid crowded and busy roads

Wear good glasses and hearing aid if needed

Carry only as much as you comfortably can

Wear a hat or cap

Carry an umbrella

Wear non-skid shoes

Use the pavement

THE BED-RIDDEN PATIENT

Patients especially elderly can be bed-redden due to fractures, a paralytic attack, a bad back, a heart attack, severe infections, or any other chronic problem. Prolonged immobilization can lead to fluid retention and oedema,(swelling) thrombophlebitis (block in leg veins), muscle wasting, pressure sores, and general decline in all functions.

To avoid these problems, bed rest should be avoided as far as possible. If the patient can be managed in a sitting or semi reclining position it is better. Frequent changes in position are also advisable. Food and drinks should never be given with the patient lying down, or it may enter the lungs and cause a condition called 'aspiration pneumonia'. Physiotherapeutic exercises should be done twice a day. Dynamic mattresses that inflate and deflate are best to prevent pressure sores. The patient must be mobilized as fast as possible. Wheel chairs, canes and other aids should be encouraged. Urinary catherisation should be avoided as far as possible since it can get infected. External catherisation in males and diapers in females may be used.

THE EIGHTY PLUS

A dilemma faced by many families is what to do when an eighty plus patient becomes serious. Should one admit him to a hospital, subject him to all sorts of investigations and intensive management OR simply leave him alone to die quietly at home? I remember a patient I was called to see in Delhi. She was a hypertensive and suffered a stroke outside the country. Her daughter, whom she had gone to help there, panicked at the potential expenses, put her on a plane and brought her to India. She was obviously in a bad state by the time she arrived. Her son and daughter-in-law cared for her day and night and when they knew the end was near, they lit a lamp but did not let me admit her or give any emergency medication and only wanted me to certify her death.

Another gentleman in his late eighties had severe pneumonia and went into respiratory failure. Due to excellent management in the ICCU, he survived and lived another five years!

A third gentleman in his mid eighties suffered a paralytic stroke and went into coma. He was admitted to ICCU and in spite of intensive multi-specialty care; he died after ten days in hospital.

Now the point is, the second gentleman in his late eighties came out of severe respiratory failure with no residual damage. If he had not been admitted, thinking it was of no use; he would not have lived another five years. Attitude of the patient also plays a major role in the decision-making, since the sort of patient who feels he is four times twenty and not eighty years of age, has to be treated differently from one who has a defeatist nature. Reacting to a young congressman who had ridiculed him on account of his old age, John Quincy Adams once remarked, "Tell that young man that an ass is older at thirty than a man at eighty!"

So when asked for advice about intensive management of an eighty plus, I leave the decision to the relatives. If the situation seems really irreversible, home care is best, with minimal intervention; but if the patient has a good constitution, with a positive attitude, and the condition is curable, I think even an eighty plus deserve the best care possible. But like I said, the decision has to be made by the family with guidance from their physician. A case of "different strokes for different folks"

Recently I had a lady patient who is 80 years of age. She simply refuses to grow old and keeps coming to me with minor nagging complaints, since she wants to maintain perfect health. Normally it would take a lot of effort on my part to convince her that a few minor complaints should be tolerated and not treated, and give her minimum possible medication; but yesterday I decided to take a different tack. I told her that she was looking particularly pretty and healthy, and what was the secret? She was absolutely delighted with the compliment and for the first time, immediately accepted that the problem she had come for was very minor and was easily satisfied with the minimal medication that I had prescribed.

Here are a few more examples of active 'young' eighty plus heroes -

Aging

At 80	Jyoti Basu was chief minister of Bengal.
At 81	Benjamin Franklin engineered the diplomacy that led to the adoption of the U.S. constitution.
At 82	Winston Churchill wrote a four-volume book 'A history of the English speaking people'
At 82	Leo Tolstoy wrote 'I cannot be silent'
At 82	Goethe finished 'Faust'
At 83	Karunanidhi again became chief minister of Tamil Nadu in India.
At 88	Pablo Casals was still giving cello concerts
At 89	Arthur Rubenstein gave one of his greatest recitals.
At 90	Pablo Picasso was still drawing and engraving.
At 90	former Indian Prime Minister Morarji Desai was still going strong.
At 90	famous painter MF Husain was still painting (unfortunately we lost him recently!)
At 91	Eamon De Valera was still serving as President of Ireland.
At 93	George Bernard Shaw wrote 'Far fetched fables'
At 100	Grandma Moses was still painting!

Although most of these celebrities had already attained fame and fortune, they continued to lead productive lives and never became 'old'!

In the last chapter, we are going to talk about death, since it is the final act before the curtain falls.

✦ ✦ ✦ ✦

Part – V

Death
A Problem for All

34

Death and Euthanasia
(The Final Curtain)

There is a reaper whose name is death, and with his sickle keen,
He reaps the bearded grain at a breath,
And the flowers which grow between."
Longfellow.

Death is a great enigma, which has troubled us since the world began. Man has taken giant strides towards advancement and civilization, since the Stone Age – but death still remains an unsolved riddle. Children have troubled their parents from time immemorial with the eternal question –" what is death, and what comes after it", philosophers have puzzled over it, writers have written volumes on it and poets have eulogised it –

" Tell me not in mournful numbers,
Life is but an empty dream;
For the soul is dead that slumbers,
And things are not what they seem;
Life is real, life is earnest,
And the grave is not its goal,
Dust thou art to dust returnest,
Was not spoken of thy soul. "

W. Longfellow

Death is a problem for physicians, lawyers, theologians, transplants surgeons and last but not the least - the layman. It is a sword hanging perpetually over our heads – and the thread by which it is suspended is very slender – no one knows when this thread will break and the sword descend mercilessly. It is this *uncertainty* that makes us most afraid of it.

In simple words – "death is the cessation of activity of all the vital functions of the body- nervous, respiratory and circulatory." When a person is dying, due to a failing circulation or respiration – he can be kept alive by artificial means – and he may survive if his normal functions resume.

If his organs are needed for transplantation, he can be kept "alive" in this way till the necessary organ is removed from his body; but once the resuscitative measures are stopped, the person will surely die. The question that arises here is, when did the person die, and what was the cause of death, respiratory or circulatory? The time of death also cannot be ascertained, as the person had been kept alive by artificial means at a time when he was *dying but not dead.* This could well entail a legal problem Courts also require the precise time and nature of death in the settlement of manslaughter charges, inheritance claims, insurance procedures, tax problems and disposition of jointly held money and property. A typical example is of a couple, who were involved in a car accident. The husband died immediately – but the wife remained in a state of coma for 17 days during which time she was artificially maintained. The husband's will decreed that if his wife survived him, all his money went to her, if not, all his money went to a "distant cousin" The lawyer for the "distant cousin" contended that both the husband and wife died together, as they both lost their "power to act" together. But the court invalidated their claim saying that the wife's beating heart during the days of coma delayed her death by 17 days.

Theologians too feel they have a say in the matter. They may think it sinful for a doctor to interfere with death by means of resuscitative measures and then to withdraw them when he knows that it is going to be of no use. But they must remember and adhere to the ancient, unwritten and usually unspoken pact between a good doctor and his patient - A doctor backed by his training, experience and entire history of medicine has but one aim – to do what he can, within the law, for every individual under his care. Only *he* has the perspective to declare when it is best to stop all resuscitative measures and let a man die in natural course of time – of course the final decision being taken with the consent of the patient's family, who must be completely satisfied that their relative cannot live again. In this modern era, there are various ways and means of detecting the time, cause and confirmation of death -

1. When the EEG (electro encephalogram or brain waves) becomes Iso electric (flat). Statisticians have proved that once the EEG becomes Iso-electric, the patient cannot survive for more than 5 days. Therefore it is inhumane and useless to maintain the patient on a mechanical respirator.

2. Patient should be totally unaware of and unresponsive to his surroundings – so that even the most painful stimulus evokes no vocal or other response – not even a groan, withdrawal of limb or quickening of respiration.

3. Patient should be observed for at least one hour to make sure that there are no muscular movements of spontaneous respiration.

4. All reflexes should be absent.

5. Pupil should be dilated and unresponsive. All these tests should be repeated 24 hours later and show no changes for the final confirmation unless resuscitation is carried out within this period.

Until recently the definition of death was based on there being a boundary drawn between life and death, by the final heart beat or the last breath. But today the concept has shifted more to brain death. Both respiration and circulation can be restored – thanks to various resuscitative measures including portable respirators, defibrillators, external and internal cardiac massage, electrical pace makers, heart surgery, angioplasty, and use of thrombolytic treatment, but once brain death sets in – it is irreversible. When respiration and circulation cease, vital nerve cells in the brain are denied oxygen, and will die within 3-8 minutes, if resuscitation is not carried out.

A person can be made to survive in a "vegetative" state for years; if his lungs and heart are normally maintained by external means and needs of his body are satisfied through tubes – as long as his brain is healthy. In this context the notable example is of Lie Daganais, a 21-year-old woman from Montreal who met with a car accident. She remained in a state of coma for 12 years, after which she succumbed without regaining consciousness. She was maintained for those 12 years on artificial respiratory and other devices.

Since a long time, man has been trying to conquer death. He has learnt to combat respiratory and circulatory failures, up to a point, but brain death still remains an insurmountable mountain. He has started climbing this mountain too since recent experiments have proved that brain cells can be grown outside the body, and then transplanted within it, but the pinnacle is still not in sight. When man does manage to conquer death, the words of W. Longfellow will come true -

"Then ye shall strike at death,

And when death is indeed dead;

Then ye shall be immortal".

P A S AND EUTHANASIA (MERCY KILLING)

There is a lot of interest in mercy killing these days, as the population of the world is increasingly aging. So let us try to understand what euthanasia is, and its current status.

An adult who is mentally competent can normally accept or reject a mode of treatment suggested by a doctor, and this choice of the patient has to be honoured by the physician.

Physician Assisted Suicide **(PAS)** or euthanasia or mercy-killing is an act wherein, *at the request of a competent, terminally ill patient, a physician provides the necessary medical means, and the required instructions, to help him to commit suicide or take his own life.*

V A E on the other hand, is Voluntary Active Euthanasia, *where a physician at the request of a competent patient mercifully kills him by administering a lethal dose of drug.*

Voluntary Passive Euthanasia

Here a physician terminates the life sustaining support system at the request of a terminally ill patient, who then dies. But the doctor can refuse to comply with the patient's request, as there is no binding on him to do so.

Is Euthanasia or Physician Assisted Suicide legal?

The Indian perspective:

Most doctors get queries from patients especially the aged and the terminally ill whether their life can be ended so that they can escape the torture that their existence has now become. As of today, in India, mercy killing is illegal although various groups especially from the state of Kerala are actively petitioning in favour of it. Even for cutting off life support systems at the request of the patient or relatives, the law is not very clear. Mumbai High Court, in Ku. Pranjali Vs.Chief Secretary, Union of India and others, 2000, was petitioned seeking permission to receive mercy killing, through her mother, as the petitioner was only 10 years of age. Pranjali was suffering from a serious ailment, and not responding to any kind of treatment given to her. She therefore sought permission for mercy killing to end her agony and also because she was unable to continue to meet her medical expenses. The court's reply was "In view of constitutional rights as to life, permission for mercy killing cannot be granted to the petitioner. She later passed away. In view of age Kumari Pranjali, is quite incompetent to make up her mind, and for this kind of sensitive issue the mother may not be able to take a decision on behalf of her child.2) In view of the financial difficulty, as the family members are not in a position to afford adequate and appropriate medical care, the court passed relevant orders instructing the state to provide the required medical care.

There is also the poignant story of Vishwanath who was a paraplegic. When he was dying of a terminal problem he wanted to donate his organs so that it could help many people, but unfortunately the courts did not give permission for euthanasia, and by the time he died, his organs were not fit for donation. His grieving mother is working for the handicapped, and actively campaigning for euthanasia.

 We have all heard of the unfortunate case of Aruna Shanbaug who had been molested by a ward boy and left to live a vegetative life for 37 years. The petition for her mercy killing was recently rejected by the courts citing the reason that she was still responsive and did not meet most of the criteria to be labeled a permanent vegetative. She later passed away naturally. In a path-breaking judgment, the Supreme Court allowed "passive euthanasia" of *withdrawing life support to patients in permanently vegetative state (PVS) but rejected outright active euthanasia of ending life through administration of lethal substances.*

The court decreed that in a case where a request for euthanasia was made, a panel of three doctors must first certify that the patient was to all practical purposes in a vegetative state from which there was absolutely no chance of recovery. Armed with this, the courts have to be approached and after receiving the orders, they could proceed with the mercy killing. The punishment for illegal mercy killing as of today in India is either imprisonment for life or imprisonment up to 10 years with fine or both.

The first country to legalise Euthanasia, was Australia where it became effective in 1996. Bob Dent, a farmer suffering from incurable cancer was the first person on whom a computer-controlled machine was used to deliver a lethal dose of a drug. The conditions for Euthanasia in Australia are:

The attending physician must be convinced about the patient's decision being totally voluntary. He must further be convinced that the illness is untreatable and certify that the patient is suffering from unacceptable pain or suffering. The diagnosis has to be confirmed by a second physician, plus a doctor trained in palliative care (one who relieves pain). A psychiatrist must also evaluate and certify that the patient is of sound mind. A cooling period of 7 days is mandatory, and the person must wait for another 2 days after the final decision is taken. A computerised system enables a fatal injection to be administered to the patient without the doctor being actively involved. *The bill however has been challenged in court.*

In Oregon USA, "death with dignity" act had been passed by ballot in 1994. Here an adult resident of Oregon can request his physician for a prescription, which will help him to terminate his own life. The waiting or cooling period here is 15 days. Otherwise the parameters are same as those in Australia. The law however never became effective as *in 1995 it was challenged in court and a judge found it unconstitutional.* Terri Schiavo's case received a lot of media attention. She became brain dead about 15 years back due to a metabolic deficiency that lasted for 6-10 minutes after her heart stopped beating. Since then she had been maintained on tube feeding which was removed and re-inserted thrice on petitioning and counter petitioning by her husband and her parents. Ultimately on 31ˢᵗ of March 2005 she passed away when her tube feeding had been withdrawn for more than 13 days.

Netherlands is the only country where not only is P A S legal, but is also widely practiced. In the last 14 years 4.5% of hospital deaths have been physician assisted. There have been protests of involuntary PAS being carried out on children, vegetative patients and mentally incompetent, which is said to be up to 0.8% of all hospital deaths.

In the U.K., euthanasia is totally illegal and is regarded as murder.

So you see, euthanasia is still a raging controversy and until such time that it becomes legal, doctors like me can only reassure and counsel patients, especially one of them who rings me up every 3 months or so and queries - "Hello! I am your first prospective euthanasia patient, has it been legalized yet?"

REFERENCES :

1.   **Koch KA.** The language of death Euthanatos et mors – The science of understanding (Review) Critical Care Clinics 1996;52: 386-93

2.   **Blandon RJ, Szalay US.** Should physicians aid their patients in dying? The public perspective, JAMA 1992; 267:2658-62.

3.   **Emanuel EJ, Fairclough DL, Daniels ER, et al.** Euthanasia and physician assisted suicide: attitudes and experiences of oncology patients oncologists and the public. Lancet 1996; 347: 1805-10.

4.   **Caralis PV, Hammond JS.** Attitudes of medical

students house staff and faculty physicians towards euthanasia and termination of life sustaining treatment. Crit Care Med 1992; 20:683-90

5. **Meisel A**. The right to die, 2nd Ed. New York: John Wiley and Sons. 1995.

6. **Gert B, Culver CM**. Distinguishing between active and passive euthanasia. Clin Geriatr Med 1986; 2:29-36.

7. **Paalegrino ED**. Doctors must not kill. J Clin Ethics 1992;3 : 95-109

Quill TE. Doctor I want to die – will you help me? JAMA

Comments and Commends

'This book is good and concise reading material for those who wish to lead a long and stress free life. Worth having such a prized knowledge base in every home.'

Padmashree Smt. Lila Poonawalla

- Chairperson Alpha Laval

'Dr. Geeta Sundar, MD, an astute Physician, in this step-by-step presentation, has shown us the way for effecting a change in our lifestyle for a healthier life. This book is a compulsory read for all those who wish to keep their mind on an even keel and maintain a healthy heart'.

Dr. M Durairaj

- Cardiologist

-former Physician to the President of India

'This book is a multidisciplinary guide to health distilled from the rich experience of a quintessential doctor who believes in a holistic approach with minimal medication in treating the human body. It is a must read.'

Dr. OP Chawla

- Ex-Director

National institute of Bank
Management and Currently financial advisor.

Books Written By the Author

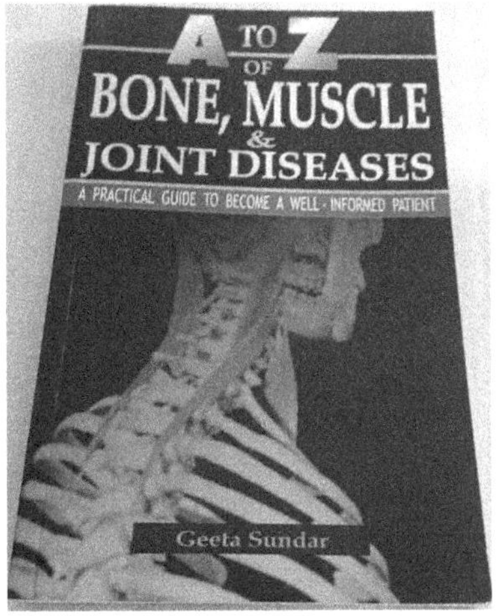

Macmillan A-Z of Bone Muscle and Joint Diseases—Bestseller

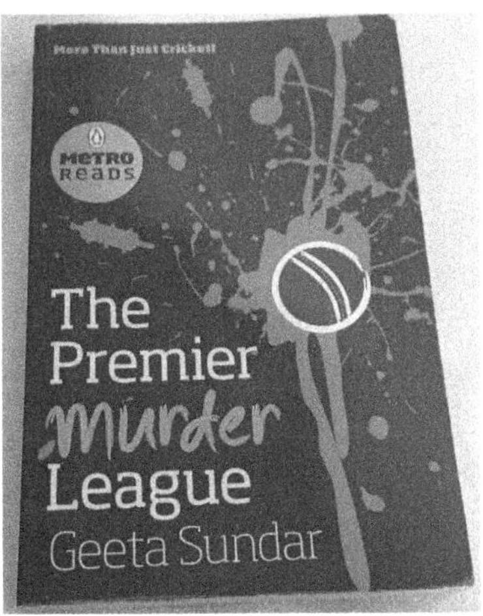

Penguin Premier Murder League—Murder Mystery T-20 Novel

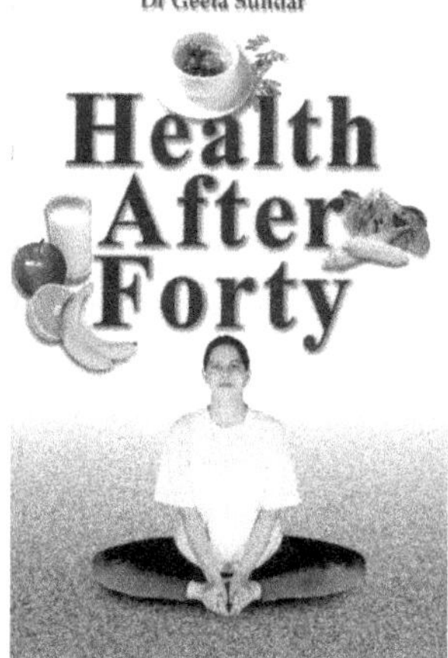

Macmillan Health After Forty—Bestseller

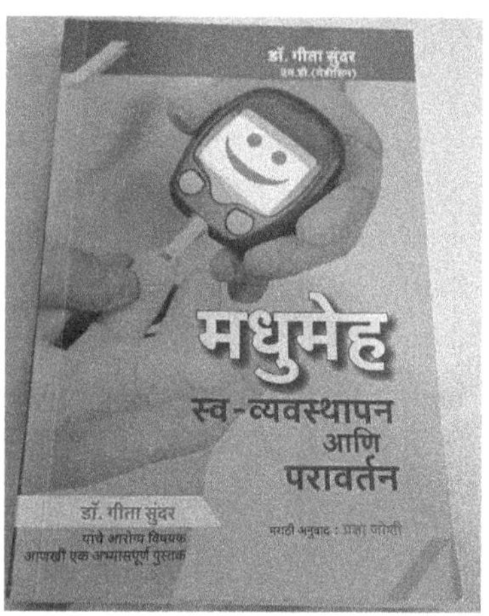

Becoming Shakespeare Madhumeha—Sva-vyavassthapan aaniparavartan (Marathi)

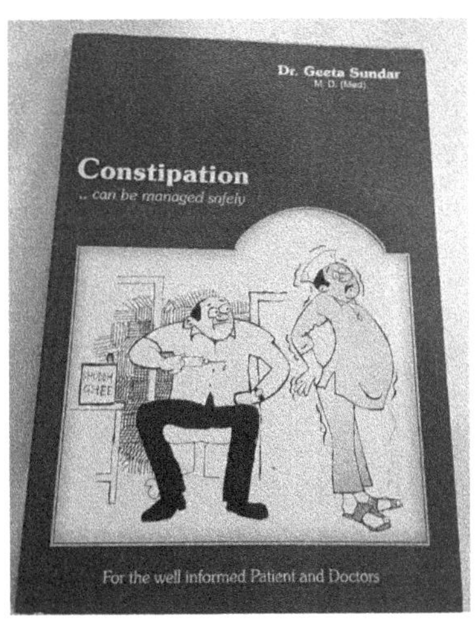

Amazon US Constipation Can Be Managed Safely

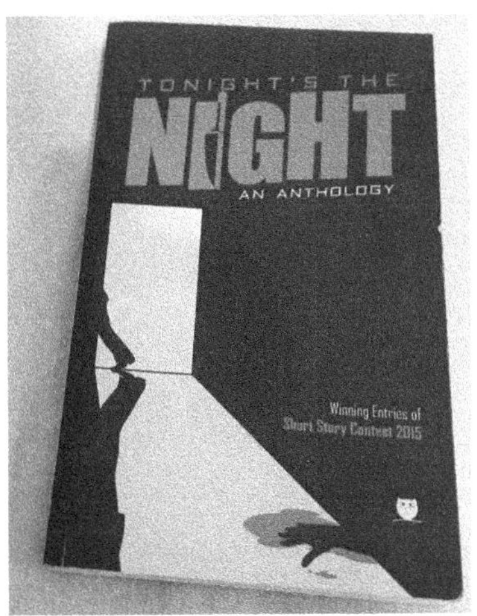

Notionpress TONIGHT'S The Night—Collection of Prize-winning Short Stories By Many Authors

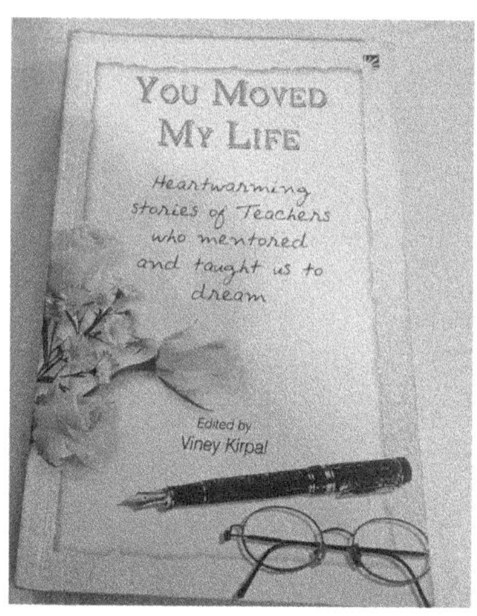

Sterling You Moved My Life—Collection of Articles on Teachers By Many Famous People

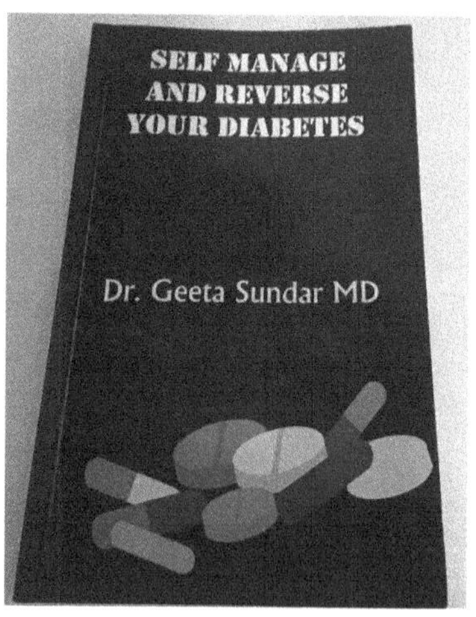

Becoming Shakespeare Self-Manage and Reverse Your Diabetes

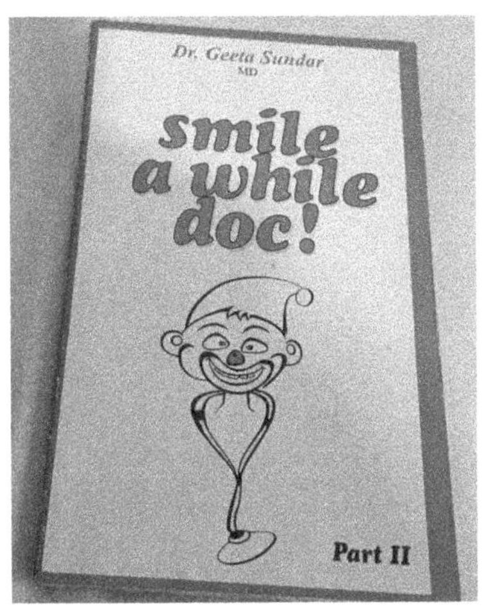

Self Published—Funny Incidents from Doctors Lives.

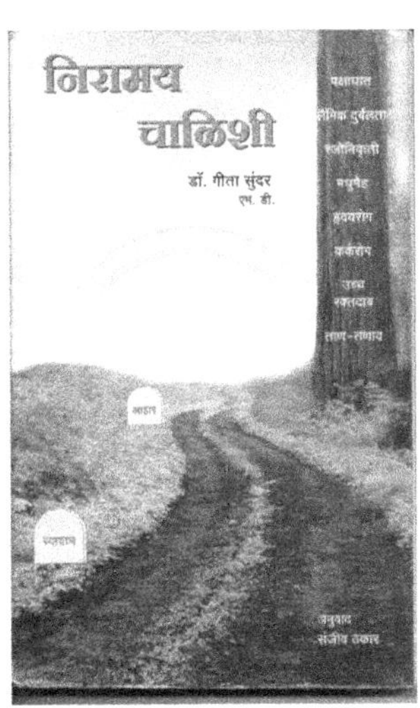

Macmillan Niramaya Chalishi in Marathi

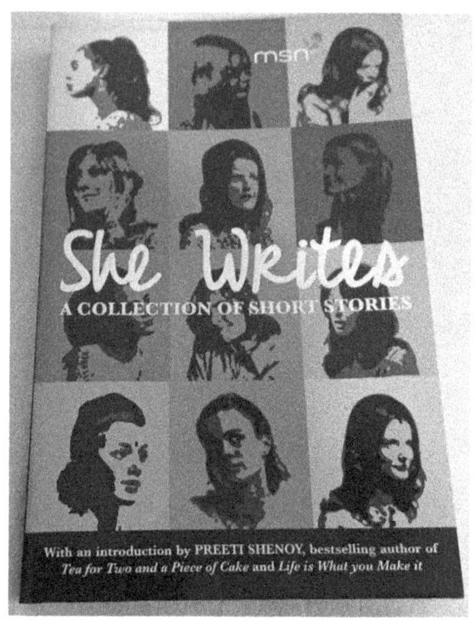

Random House She Writes—Collection of Prize Winning Storiesby 11 Authors

www.ingramcontent.com/pod-product-compliance
Lightning Source LLC
Chambersburg PA
CBHW041302120726
48005CB00014B/1838